THE SIMPLE MEDITERRANEAN DIET

Easy Steps to Change Your Diet

...And Change Your Life

ARIEL SOFFER, MD

Cardiologist and Creator of SimpleMD

"To my patients over the last 25 years,

thanks for allowing me into your lives!"

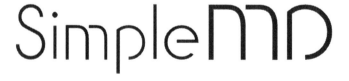

Printed in the United States of America

ISBN: 978-0-9974513-0-6

Table of Contents

Acknowledgements

NO USEFUL BODY OF WORK is done in isolation. My 36-year-journey from pre-med college to medical school, residency, fellowship, academic, and private practice have led me to here. I would not have been able to make the journey without my loving parents for their nurturing love and direction. My mother Mina Soffer and I collaborated on our first book on Mitral Valve Prolapse, and she showed me the importance of perseverance and the importance of clarifying difficult subjects for patients. My father Gad Soffer, as a university professor and academic, helped me to be prolific and studious as well as to balance it all with equal parts of fun and excitement.

A proper "thank you" could not be complete without my brother and sister Avi and Emira, who have always supported my efforts and been there for useful critique and helpful suggestions. Of course, I cannot forget my wife, my queen, my "Malka" (Maria Soffer). Her eternal optimism and consistent way of being has allowed me to pursue my life's work. Our kids Evan and Shayna have kept me motivated to try and make the world a more knowledgeable and better place to live.

Professionally, this project could not have been completed with out the following instrumental colleagues and friends. First and foremost is Dr. Sasson Moulavi, who has paved the way for so many with his relentless pursuit of weight management and wellness strategies. Also, Adam Kustin's creative spirit has encouraged me to continue on this path and to be able to reach so many people. Dr. Marc Weinberg has been a great sounding board and his passion for healthful nutrition inspires me. Tainet Gonzalez my assistant has been a loyal and lovely addition to our lives well into our second decade together. Cecila Pernas, A.R.N.P, Maryanne Martinez, P.A.-C, Nicolette Tabacco, RDCS, and Dr. Yael Myers, and Dr. Neil Furman have been great clinical sounding boards for me.

Of course Jon VanZile's ability to edit my thoughts regarding the Mediterranean Diet and put them in such a "Simple" way has been so very helpful to the SimpleMD concept.

I also wanted to thank Dr. Mehmet Oz, who I first met on my ABC News segment in Miami. His body of work both in the national media and in the cardiovascular space has inspired me to try to reach others beyond the scope of our individual practices.

Mostly, I wanted to thank the thousands of patients that have allowed me to be a part of their lives through the years. They have taught me so much by letting me into their lives, sometimes in their most vulnerable moments, and the privilege will never be forgotten.

Foreword

AS A BARIATRIC DOCTOR who deals with overweight and obese patients, the Mediterranean Diet has been a great asset in helping them achieve a healthy weight and reduce many health risks.

Dr. Ariel Soffer's book offers a concise, fact-filled blueprint that gets to the point and is supported by relevant, sound science. It is easy to follow, and I will be recommending his book and supporting SimpleMD products to my patients.

Dr. Soffer has had unique perspective; he is an American who was raised by parents from the Mediterranean region, and he is a board-certified cardiologist who knows the ravages of our typical American diet. By advocating the Mediterranean Diet for his patients, as well as using it for his own family for years, he not only preaches it but he lives it. He also greatly enlightened the medical community and me with his many lectures, talks, and TV appearances about the important benefits of extra virgin olive oil (EVOO) and red wine.

Dr. Soffer has made it easier for doctors and patients alike to live the Mediterranean lifestyle by joining forces with American Institute of Baking certified bakers, using the best extra virgin olive oil, the best red wine, and the best Mediterranean Diet ingredients to produce protein bars that are so healthful and delicious they have become a daily staple in my and many of my colleagues' diets.

If you get a chance to hear him speak on TV, tune in—or go on YouTube and view some of his lectures. And if you like this book, let your friends know, as it could make such a difference in their lives. It has in mine.

If you are overweight or suffer from elevated cholesterol or at elevated risk of heart disease, I urge you to change your eating habit and go Mediterranean. This book and the SimpleMD way may be all you ever need and some of the best "medicine" you can get.

Dr. Sasson Moulavi

Graduate of the fellowship program of the Obesity Medical Association

Founder of Smart For Life

Introduction

STEPHANIE WAS LIKE MANY of the patients who walk into my office. She hadn't had a heart attack or major health problem, but she was worried about it. She knew she was carrying some extra weight left over from her two pregnancies, and she had a history of high blood pressure and diabetes in her family. Recently, at age 37, she had started to experience joint and lower back pain.

Before coming in, she'd spent some time on the Internet, looking for a good diet. She'd even tried some, including Jenny Craig, Weight Watchers, and a few others. She'd given the Mediterranean Diet a try after reading about its impressive results, but it was too hard for her to make all that food from scratch every day as she tried to balance her busy family life with her job as a teacher's aide and with her health goals.

We started off like I do with all of my new patients. I asked a lot of questions about her medical history, her lifestyle, and her day-to-day life. A typical picture soon emerged. Stephanie was the cook in her household, and estimated they ate steak or hamburgers three times a week. She loved to cook with butter or margarine, and while she didn't report being under tremendous stress, she was busy every day.

After discussing her history, we did her exam and blood work. Her BMI was 33, which was considered obese on her 5'6" medium frame. Her cholesterol was high, and her blood showed evidence of chronic inflammation. Finally, her blood glucose was slightly elevated, pushing into the pre-diabetic zone.

Stephanie's story so far would be familiar to any cardiologist in America. She wasn't actively sick yet, but she was right to be worried. Like so many other

Americans, Stephanie was on the road to heart disease—the number one killer of both men and women in the United States. In most cases, doctors would suggest "lifestyle modifications" and reach for the prescription pad to scribble out a prescription or two.

But this is where Stephanie's story takes a hopeful turn—and the reason I'm writing this book. Over the past decade, it's been almost impossible to avoid the avalanche of positive research on the Mediterranean Diet. This diet is modeled after the healthy lifestyles of the Mediterranean basin. It features lots of seafood, great fruits and vegetables, whole grains, the incredibly powerful health benefits of extra virgin olive oil, and red wine in moderation. It's one of the only diets in the world that has been clinically proven to lower your risk of heart disease and other diseases, help you lose weight, and actually extend your life. Yet Stephanie's first experience with the Mediterranean Diet is common. If you've been living a pretty "normal" American life—lots of red meat and saturated fat, busy and stressed out—it can be hard to change your habits to those of a more traditional lifestyle.

This is where SimpleMD comes in. I immediately recommended that Stephanie lose weight and enrolled her in a program we call SimpleMD Rapid Weight Loss. This program takes the best of the Mediterranean Diet and makes it easy to follow by providing ready-to-eat SimpleMD protein bars made with authentic extra virgin olive oil and real red wine. Instead of spending hours and hours in the kitchen, Stephanie was soon eating five bars a day: a Greek Yogurt bar for breakfast, followed by a Caffe' Latte mid-morning snack bar, a Chocolate Almond bar for lunch, and a Chocolate Date bar for her afternoon snack. At dinner, she'd enjoy a green salad with a vinaigrette dressing made with more extra virgin olive oil and a nice piece of lean fish.

Her results were astounding. She was eating about 1,000 calories a day; she wasn't hungry and cruised through her first 30 days. Meanwhile, those extra pounds just kept dropping off. She lost 15 pounds that first month and went down two dress sizes. Her cholesterol improved and her blood glucose dropped into the normal range. After another month, she'd dropped a total of 25 pounds and hit her goal. At this point, she was confident enough to start incorporating more prepared foods into her diet again, but she stuck with the Mediterranean Diet and six months later she'd lost 42 pounds! She loved being back to her pre-pregnancy weight, and her blood work was fantastic. Last time I checked, she and her husband were planning a trip to the Mediterranean for themselves, where I hope they'll enjoy all the incredible foods the region has to offer.

As a doctor, Stephanie's results are thrilling—because they are possible for everyone. SimpleMD was created to bring the benefits of the Mediterranean Diet within reach for everyone, no matter how busy you are, whether you're an expert cook or can hardly boil water, and whether you live in Miami or Anchorage.

Remember, this is not a diet, but a lifestyle transformation! Our mission is to take the fantastic amount of recent scientific research and put it at your fingertips. Whether it is myself, our SimpleMD products, or the coaching resources on our website (www.thesimplemd.com), we want to be there for you every step of the way!

Chapter 1
Why the Mediterranean Diet
Is Better Than the Rest

IMAGINE THIS LIFE: you wake up naturally with the sun and head to your kitchen for a light breakfast consisting of coffee, perhaps with cream, and a whole-grain croissant or cereal. After breakfast, you walk or take a short bike ride to work for the morning hours and deal with your normal work issues. At lunch, you might return home for an hour or two to eat with your family, or perhaps head to a local café with coworkers, where you enjoy a salad of fresh, local vegetables tossed with vinaigrette created from pure, first-pressed local olive oil. Perhaps you have a piece of locally sourced fish as well. When your workday ends around 5 p.m., you walk or bike home for a dinner that might include a small portion of locally raised meat, such as lamb, or perhaps more fish and maybe some locally sourced goat cheese. And of course there's roasted vegetables tossed in more olive oil and another salad. You enjoy a glass of wine with dinner. Afterward, you have the evening to spend with your family or maybe taking a walk to the local plaza, then, it's off to bed.

This is exactly the kind of life people lead throughout the Mediterranean basin, including southern Spain, Italy, and even into Morocco. It's a pattern of life that operates by rhythms that are centuries old.

When doctors and health experts talk about the Mediterranean Diet, they are talking about food, of course, but it's much more than that. In reality, they are talking about the many studies showing that the type of idyllic lifestyle I just described that results in fewer diseases, a longer life, and greater overall health and happiness. It's marked by lower stress, better sleep, light or moderate daily exercise, and plenty of wholesome and excellent foods prepared with care and respect for the ingredients.

Now contrast this lifestyle with the typical American weekday experience. According to research from the Gallup polling organization, the average American gets less than the recommended 7 hours of sleep a night, so from the first bleat of the alarm clock, you start the day with a sleep deficit. Breakfast is a hurried affair, often consisting of a pastry or maybe nothing at all. Also according to Gallup, Americans work longer hours than almost any other industrialized country in the Western hemisphere. Almost 40 percent of us work more than 50 hours a week. In 2015, the average full-time employed adult worked 47 hours a week, logging hours six out of seven days.

And all this work is making our lives more stressful. In 2011, the American Psychological Association reported that, "Chronic stress is becoming a public health crisis." Almost half of Americans have reported increasing stress levels, with worries about job stability, finances, and the economy topping the list.[1]

When we're not working and stressing about money, we're eating and not getting enough exercise. According to the United States Department of Agriculture in the 2000 study "Profiling Food Consumption in America," the average American adult consumed more than 2,700 calories per day—over 35 percent more than the recommended 2,000-calories per day for an adult man. This is a whopping 24.5 percent increase from 1970.[2] Meanwhile,

---

1. "Stressed in America." American Psychological Association, http://www.apa.org/monitor/2011/01/stressed-america.aspx.

2. "Profiling Food Consumption in America." United States Department of Agriculture, http://www.usda.gov/factbook/chapter2.pdf.

according to the Centers for Disease Control and Prevention, as many as 80 percent of Americans don't get the recommended amount of exercise to maintain good health.[3]

Unfortunately, we're now seeing the effects of this accelerated, stressful, calorie-rich, and exercise-deficient lifestyle. Obesity has reached epidemic proportions. According to the National Institutes of Health, almost 70 percent of American adults are considered overweight or obese.[4] Naturally, this comes along with a host of health problems. Diabetes. Increased rates of certain cancers. Hypertension. Liver disease. And of course, heart disease, which remains the leading killer of Americans. As a cardiologist, I see it every day: patients suffering from heart disease that might have been prevented.

In a perfect world, who wouldn't prefer to live the life of Italian villager? Of course we all would. I certainly would. But here's the problem, unless you're planning to pick up stakes and relocate your family halfway around the world, it just isn't practical. So many "diet" books mean well, but when we get down to the details, they are recommending a lifestyle that is nearly impossible in today's America. You'd need to carve out five extra hours in every day for all of the sleep, exercise, and food prep time to follow the complicated plan; and when it turns out to be impossible, you'd have the added guilt and stress of "failing" another major diet.

This book and the program behind it, SimpleMD, is built on a simple idea: I want to bring the benefits of the Mediterranean Diet and lifestyle to contemporary America. I want to make it possible for you to enjoy the wonderful health benefits of a different approach to eating and life, without making unattainable demands on your time, attention, and pocketbook.

The good news? This is totally possible.

---

3. *"Exercise or Physical Activity." Centers for Disease Control and Prevention, http://www.cdc.gov/nchs/fastats/exercise.htm.*

4. *"Overweight and Obesity Statistics." National Institute of Diabetes and Digestive and Kidney Diseases,*

    http://www.niddk.nih.gov/health-information/health-statistics/Pages/overweight-obesity-statistics.aspx

MODERN AMERICAN LIFE: CHRONIC INFLAMMATION

Before I go further, I want to dig a little deeper into some of the underlying issues with the modern American diet and lifestyle. Excess calories are a problem, yes, but they aren't the only issue we'll be dealing with. In fact, researchers now understand that we are experiencing an epidemic of chronic inflammation that contributes to virtually every disease of the modern age.

Chronic inflammation is different from the kind of inflammation you experience after you get a small burn or cut. That kind of inflammation is called "acute" inflammation. It is local to the site of the injury, and it's a crucial part of the immune system response. Acute inflammation is characterized by the activation of white blood cells that rush to limit the damage caused by an injury and to start the healing process.

Chronic inflammation is a whole different, and much more dangerous, type of inflammation. To put it simply, your immune system produces chemicals that cause inflammation. When those chemicals are limited to the site of an injury, it's helpful and necessary. However, when they are produced in response to non-injuries, they are left free to rampage through your circulatory system, causing all kind of trouble.

What kinds of non-injuries are known to increase your level of inflammatory chemicals? You might have guessed already—the list includes:

- Stress
- Lack of sleep
- Excess weight (fat cells actually produce pro-inflammatory chemicals)
- Lack of adequate fiber
- Foods like sugars, simple starches, and trans-fats and saturated fats

Thousands of studies have shown that our modern lifestyles are highly pro-inflammation. No less an authority than the *Journal of the American College of Cardiology* declared that, "Western dietary patterns warm up inflammation."

HEART DISEASE AND INFLAMMATION

Nowhere is inflammation more dangerous than in your heart. Your heart receives its blood through tiny arteries called coronary arteries. When those arteries become clogged with fatty deposits and cholesterol, the blood flow to your heart is reduced. These fatty deposits are called plaque deposits. When a plaque deposit ruptures, it can send pieces of plaque showering down your coronary arteries. Just like in your household plumbing, sooner or later one of these bigger pieces will get stuck and prohibit blood from flowing through the artery. This means the heart tissue past the blockage can't receive any oxygenated blood. The result is a heart attack.

This grim pattern is repeated all too often: in fact, heart disease is the number one killer for both American men and woman.

Although we are still learning exactly how this process works, heart disease begins with chronic inflammation in the very delicate inner walls of your coronary arteries. We know that pro-inflammatory chemicals injure these delicate walls, which trigger your immune system to send white blood cells rushing to the area. The white blood cells combine with cells in your artery wall and form a fatty streak on the artery wall. Over time, lipids (fats) like cholesterol migrate to the site of the injury, and the plaque starts to form and grow. Soon a hard shell forms over the top of the plaque. This is called calcification, and it can be a very dangerous situation. Heart attacks commonly start when calcified plaque deposits break.

The scariest thing? This process—known medically as atherosclerosis—often has no symptoms. Cardiologists like myself measure a person's heart attack risk based on certain factors, like your family history of heart disease, if you smoke or not, and your weight and dietary patterns. But for many people, they have no indication that a plaque is slowly growing inside their coronary arteries.

For tens of thousands of people every year, their first indication they have serious heart disease is a fatal heart attack.

BEWARE THE FALSE DIET PROPHETS

With all of the pressing medical issues we face, it would be nice to think there was some broad agreement about how to address the problems. In fact, doctors like myself often find ourselves giving the same advice over and over: lose some weight, eat more vegetables and fiber, get good exercise and sleep, try to reduce stress as much as possible.

This is all good advice, but for many people, it's just not enough to hear and follow common sense health advice. Instead, people like to believe in the "magic bullet" health cure. You see this everywhere. Pills and programs that promise weight loss, youthful vitality, lowered disease risk, a longer life, better sex, detoxification and cleansing ... you name it, and chances are someone is out there with a specialized program for it.

This can be especially confusing because many of these programs are based on a nugget of good research, which is then expanded to a major lifestyle program. Although I don't want to spend too much time on these programs, I want to stress how they are different from the Mediterranean lifestyle I'm proposing. The Mediterranean Diet and lifestyle is based on the concept of balance. The lifestyle seeks to add balance to your life, by keeping work and stressful activities in perspective. And the diet is based on a wide array of wholesome, "whole" foods that are packed with nutrients and antioxidants. There is no secret to this program—it's based on principles that have been followed for thousands of years, studied for almost a century, and have been conclusively shown to lower your risk of disease as well as help you lose excess weight.

Let's compare it to some of the most popular diet programs out there.

THE ATKINS / LOW-CARB DIETS

For many people, the word "diet" itself has become almost synonymous with the type of low-carb diet championed by Dr. Robert Atkins in his best-selling books *Dr. Atkins Diet Revolution* (1972) and *Dr. Atkins New Diet Revolution* (1990). There are a few variations of this diet, including *The Zone* and *The South Beach Diet*, but they all operate on the same basic idea.

According to this approach, the human body was biologically engineered over tens of thousands of years to eat based on the environment we lived in. This meant lots of protein, because early and prehistoric humans were hunter/gatherers who lived on fresh meat as often as possible; and few sweets, which were rare and difficult to obtain.

Over time, however, people got good at producing simple and cheap carbohydrates. At first this just meant refined grains like white flour, but in recent decades, it has also meant a flood of cheap, highly caloric sugar in the form of high fructose corn syrup. Suddenly, people were consuming *most* of their calories from these sources of carbohydrates.

From a biological point of view, this focus on simple carbs wreaks havoc with the human metabolism. All food you eat is broken down in the stomach and digestive tract, and then the nutrients are absorbed into the bloodstream. Simple carbohydrates, like sugar, are absorbed much faster than others and are almost immediately available to be used by the body as fuel. The hormone responsible for "clearing" the bloodstream of carbohydrates is insulin, and insulin control is central to low-carb diets.

With so much fuel floating around the bloodstream, the body has to produce high levels of insulin to clear the blood of all that sugar—and whatever isn't cleared fast enough is stored as extra fat. Moreover, this type of diet—high blood sugar, followed by a surge of insulin, then a "crash" in blood sugar and insulin—had been linked to multiple diseases and health problems, especially diabetes and obesity.

Low-carb diets are based on the idea that if you restrict these simple carbohydrates, your body will produce less insulin and instead be forced to burn up your fat stores for fuel. In fact, many of them feature an "induction period" at the beginning of the diet in which you restrict your intake of carbohydrates to almost zero, instead of relying on protein and fats. The idea is to trick your body into a state called *ketosis*. Basically, this means that your body stops relying on carbohydrates for fuel and instead burns fat.

It's been interesting to see the evolution of the low-carb diets since they first took America by storm in the early 1990s. Back then, "low-carb" diets were often seen as a green light to eat as much meat as you wanted. It wasn't uncommon to read about diet programs that allowed almost daily consumption of fatty red and cured meats. As long as it wasn't a carb, it was considered OK.

Since then, we've learned a lot more about the different *types* of dietary fats, and the low-carb diet gurus have changed their tune a little bit. Today, low-carb diets like the Atkins plan stresses healthy fats, like olive oil and the fats found in fish. They also stress eating lots of healthy vegetables and limiting intake of red meat. If this sounds familiar, it should—low-carb diets are starting to sound more and more like the Mediterranean Diet!

That said, the most important consideration for any diet plan is, "Does it work?" And here's where low-carb diets have a bit of a problem. First, it's not entirely clear they work, at least for the reasons proponents say they work. It's true that most people will lose weight by following a low-carb diet plan to the letter. But if you were to try this at home, what you'd soon discover is that the most popular low-carb diet plans are *also* low-calorie diet plans. Of course it's not really surprising that people will lose weight when they cut calories.

But it raises a good question: if you're going to cut calories to lose weight, does it make sense to radically cut carb calories? Are people losing weight because they are eating fewer calories, or because they are eating dramatically fewer carbs specifically? And do they keep the weight off?

First, it's important to note that there is actually very limited scientific data on low-carb diets. And what good data there is isn't encouraging when it comes to losing weight and keeping it off. In a randomized trial comparing popular weight loss plans over 18 months, the low-carb Atkins plan ranked dead last for weight loss among participants who actually finished the program. On the good side, participants did have lower cholesterol, insulin, and levels of inflammatory chemicals—but it appeared that was related to weight loss in general, not to the low-carb diet. This study was published in the prestigious Journal of the American Medical Association (JAMA).[5]

There are plenty of other studies showing the same thing—poor long-term results—but my point isn't to pick on one diet plan.[6] Instead, I'd rather point out *why* I think these types of diets fail in the long term. In the most basic terms, low-carb diets are known as *diets of exclusion*. In other words, these diets rely on cutting out

5. Dansinger ML, Gleason JA, Griffith JL, Selker HP, Schaefer EJ. Comparison of the Atkins, Ornish, Weight Watchers, and Zone diets for weight loss and heart disease risk reduction: a randomized trial. JAMA. 2005 Jan 5;293(1):43-53.

6. Foster GD, Wyatt HR, Hill JO, McGuckin BG, Brill C, Mohammed BS, Szapary PO, Rader DJ, Edman JS, Klein S. A randomized trial of a low-carbohydrate diet for obesity. N Engl J Med. 2003 May 22;348(21):2082-90.

a whole food group. I'll explain the food groups in greater detail in the next chapter, but it's enough here to note that it's almost never a good idea to exclude an entire food group, including carbohydrates.

The truth is that people *should* be eating carbs. When Dr. Atkins himself was asked to explain why so many people dropped the low-carb lifestyle he advocated, he blamed it on "carbohydrate addiction," as if bread and pasta were drugs like heroin. To me, that's dangerous thinking, and as the studies have shown, it's not sustainable over the long term.

By contrast, the Mediterranean Diet includes carbs, but it relies on the principle of balance. Of course you should be eating carbs—and they should be a delicious and wholesome part of your diet.

PALEO DIETS

Paleo Diets are a more recent version of the traditional low-carb diet. The principle behind these diets is appealing and simple. According to their supporters, humans evolved millennia ago to eat and live a certain way. Back in ancient times, they say, people were always on the move, getting near constant exercise from running and walking. Their diet was comprised mostly of protein in the form of animal products, with some fats from organ meats mixed in. Carbs were relatively rare because they had to be foraged.

According to this theory, we ran into trouble when people invented agriculture and settled down into towns and cities. Pretty quickly, we started growing massive amounts of cereal grains, like barley and wheat, and the human diet shifted from mostly protein and animal fats to mostly carbs. The result? A radical decline in human health and the introduction of previously unknown diseases, including and especially heart disease.

The so-called "paleo diet" is designed to return people to their ancestral diet. It means lots of lean proteins, healthy fats, and very few carbs of any variety. If it sounds a little bit like a repackaged low-carb diet, that's because it is.

There are a few interesting facts that seem to support this type of diet, like the fact that ancient humans did appear to grow taller before the development of agriculture (assuming that height is a measure of overall nutrition and health). But there are many more problems with it, beginning with the fact that research is increasingly disproving the basic idea behind the paleo diet. In fact, it turns out that heart disease and other "modern" diseases were relatively common among ancient humans. To prove this, a group of researchers recently subjected hundreds of mummies from four ancient civilizations: Peru, Egypt, southwestern United States, and the Aleutian Islands, to whole-body CT scans. Guess what they found? As many as 34 percent of these ancient humans showed evidence of atherosclerosis. Writing in the prestigious medical journal *The Lancet*, they concluded, "Atherosclerosis was common in these four preindustrial populations, including preagricultural hunter-gatherers."[7]

So much for eating like a caveman and living longer.

LOW-FAT DIETS

Low-fat diets were one of the original diet fads, going back decades. They've mostly been replaced in the popular imagination by the low-carb diets, but there is a point

7. Thompson RC, Allam AH, Lombardi GP, Wann LS, Sutherland ML, Sutherland JD, Soliman MA, Frohlich B, Mininberg DT, Monge JM, Vallodolid CM, Cox SL, Abd el-Maksoud G, Badr I, Miyamoto MI, el-Halim Nur el-Din A, Narula J, Finch CE, Thomas GS. Atherosclerosis across 4000 years of human history: the Horus study of four ancient populations. Lancet. 2013 Apr 6;381(9873):1211-22.

I want to make about low-fat diets. Back when doctors were advising people to eat less fat to lose weight, it's fair to say we didn't really understand how dietary fat works. After all, it seemed simple. You want to lose fat, eat less fat. There was little recognition that some fats, like omega-3 fatty acids found in cold water fish and the monounsaturated fats found in extra virgin olive oil, are actually healthy. I'll discuss this is greater depth in the next chapter, but cutting these fats out actually *raises* your risk of heart disease and *increases* inflammation.

Unfortunately, the simple "no fat" message led people to cut out all types of fat—yet another diet of exclusion based on deprivation. And it backfired spectacularly. It turned out that people who cut fat calories often substituted them with calories from simple carbohydrates. This spawned an entire industry of "low fat" food products that were actually loaded with sugar. And what happens when you eat too much sugar? It's converted into fat.

WHY IS THE MEDITERRANEAN DIET DIFFERENT?

My point is that diets of exclusion are almost never a good idea, unless you're under the medical supervision of a doctor who specifically recommends avoiding certain food groups. No matter what you hear on talk shows or read in the latest fitness magazine, there isn't a "magic metabolic bullet" that can "trick" your body into shedding weight and reducing your disease risk. This means you can skip the pills, the potions, the complicated eating programs, the fad diets, and the latest "wonder" supplement harvested from a rare fruit that only grows in the depths of the Amazonian rain forest.

So what should you do? Well, let's take a look at what the research says.

Back in 2004, an explorer named Dan Buettner traveled around the world for the National Geographic Society to study populations of very long-lived people.

He had already identified a few of these "hot spots" of longevity in Sardinia, Italy; Okinawa, Japan; and certain parts of California. Over the next few years, Buettner and his team would identify other spots in Costa Rica and Greece. He called these areas Blue Zones. The Blue Zones were characterized by a few things:

- A very high percentage of both men and women living to 100 years of age
- Very low incidence of heart disease
- Very low incidence of cancer

While Buettner went on to publish a best-selling book, it's worth noting a few things about the people who lived in the Blue Zones. People who lived in these regions generally ate diets that were high in plant material and healthy fats, with moderate alcohol consumption. They got more exercise. And they were generally more spiritual and happier.

It's no surprise to me that two of these regions are in the Mediterranean Basin, and the rest all share profound similarities with the Mediterranean lifestyle. These people are living proof that the Mediterranean Diet and the Mediterranean lifestyle really work to help people live long, with less disease, and maintain better overall health.

Buettner is far from the only researcher to reach these same conclusions. If you enter the search term "Mediterranean Diet" into the U.S. National Library of Medicine's database of peer-reviewed studies, you get more than 4,000 results. There are literally hundreds of high-quality, peer-reviewed studies showing that following the simple principles I describe in this book can benefit every area of your life. You'll lose weight, lower your disease risk, live longer, and be happier. Perhaps even better, you won't feel like you're suffering or denying yourself. To the contrary, the SimpleMD program is based on simple, scientifically validated ideas that I've worked hard to translate into a program that anyone can follow.

In the next chapter, we'll dig deeper into what your body needs to thrive—and how the average American diet is failing us all.

Chapter 2
Step One:
The Simple Foundation
of a Healthy Diet

GOOD NUTRITION IS ESSENTIAL to a healthy, long life.

This is a pretty simple statement, so it can be surprising how much confusion exists over what "good nutrition" really is. Some of this confusion is related to legitimate issues with conducting nutrition research. In the world of medical research, the "gold standard" of studies is known as a double-blind, placebo-controlled study. In this kind of study, subjects are split into two groups. The first group is the control group, meaning they do not receive the medication or therapy but instead receive a sugar pill or fake therapy. The second group is the study group. Ideally, the study subjects have no idea which group they're in. This allows scientists to compare results from both groups and come up with objective, provable results.

In the world of nutrition, unfortunately, this type of study is virtually impossible. After all, who wants to be locked away in a lab somewhere for weeks or months while they are fed only certain foods? And even if you could find people willing to do this, most of the effects of diet are long-term and take years to measure.

This means that it's very hard to actually get good data on nutrition. Scientists rely on a number of approaches, none of which are perfect. They use surveys (and we all know that people don't always tell the truth when they're asked about their diets!), and they use the kind of population studies I discussed in Chapter 1.

The second source of confusion over healthy nutrition has to do with profit motives. The sad fact is, there are a lot of snake-oil salespeople out there, pushing magical pills or supplements, or signing people up to expensive services, that may or may not be based on sound science. The popularity of these shady products only proves my central point in writing this book: there is a huge thirst for good information that can help people lose weight and prevent chronic disease.

This is what led me to the Mediterranean Diet in the first place, and what keeps me motivated to make it accessible for everyone.

In this chapter, we're going to explore the building blocks of a healthy diet. Hopefully, by the end of the chapter, you'll have a basic understanding of what your body needs to thrive—and why our food culture can be so dangerous.

MACRONUTRIENTS: PARTNERS IN HEALTH

I want to start with a simple observation: the way *you* think about food and the way *your body* thinks about food might be dramatically different. To you, food might be about flavor, companionship, comfort, family, fun, and lots of other emotionally driven things.

To your body, food is fuel and construction material.

We typically divide food into two large groups: macronutrients and micro-nutrients. If you think about food like your body does, macronutrients are the floor, walls, and ceiling of your building, while micronutrients are the fixtures, plumbing, and wiring. You need both, but in different quantities.

When it comes to macronutrients, there are three types, and they form the foundation of every diet:

Carbohydrates. We talked a bit about carbohydrates in Chapter 1, but I want to dig a little deeper into what carbohydrates are exactly and how they fit into the Mediterranean lifestyle. An easy way to think of carbs is to think of them as energy. When you eat a carbohydrate, it is converted into glucose, which is the form of sugar that the body uses for energy. There are two kinds of carbs that fall into this category:

○ *Simple carbohydrates.* These include sugar, high fructose corn syrup, honey, and other carbohydrates. These are called simple because they are easily broken down by the body and result in higher levels of blood sugar (glucose). In general, simple carbs are not a nutritious choice, because they often have little nutrient value and result in a quick burst of energy, followed by a crash. These types of carbs have also been implicated in America's ongoing obesity epidemic, especially the high fructose corn syrup found in so many soda drinks. Most nutrition experts advise people to stay away from any beverages containing high fructose corn syrup, and for good reason: these drinks are nothing but empty calories that wreak havoc with your metabolism- and are directly related to weight gain. Any extra calories you consume as simple carbohydrates and that aren't needed for immediate energy are stored as fat.

○ *Complex carbohydrates.* These are the carbs that form the foundation of the Mediterranean diet. The body also breaks down complex carbs into glucose, but because it is a more complex molecule, the breakdown takes much longer. Also, complex carbs are often packaged with yet another form of carbohydrate—fiber—that slows down the glucose absorption into your bloodstream even more. The result is lower "spikes" in your blood sugar levels, feeling fuller after a meal, and no post-carb crash. Examples of complex carbs include whole grains like oatmeal, vegetables, and most whole fruits. These complex carbohydrates form the basis of the Mediterranean diet, which is great news because they are also delicious!

Fats. Dietary fats are one of the most misunderstood of any macronutrient, thanks in part to misguided advice from nutrition experts and even government health agencies for years. Until relatively recently, all fats were lumped together into one big category, and people were told to avoid eating them. In truth, we now understand there are different *kinds* of fats, and some of them are absolutely essential to health.

- O *Saturated fats.* These are the types of fats found in red meat and animal products, full-fat dairy, and some cooking oils. Saturated fats have been linked to higher cholesterol, increased risk of heart disease and stroke, inflammation, and certain types of cancers. These fats should be eaten sparingly.
- O *Trans fats.* These types of fats are the real bad guys. Trans fats are not naturally occurring. Food producers invented them as a way to stabilize liquid vegetable oils through a process called hydrogenation (hence the term "hydrogenated fat"). These fats are very dangerous and have no health benefits. They have been linked to increased risk of heart attack, stroke, diabetes, atherosclerosis, and a host of other health issues. Because of recent changes in food labeling laws, food producers now have to list trans fats on the nutrition facts panel. Look for them, and avoid them.

O **Unsaturated fats.** This final type of fat is often called "good fat." Unsaturated fats include polyunsaturated and monounsaturated fats. This group includes the polyunsaturated fats omega-3 and omega-6 fatty acids, which can be found in cold-water fish. Monounsaturated fats are found in plant-based foods, including nuts and seeds, as well as olive oil. All of these fats are healthy and have been shown to protect your heart from heart disease, reduce inflammation, reduce the risk of certain cancers, and even reduce your risk of cognitive diseases like Alzheimer's disease. They are used throughout the body, including in the cell walls and have been shown to help remove harmful cholesterol from your arteries. The Mediterranean Diet and lifestyle relies heavily on these fats, especially extra virgin olive oil. I'll talk more about this later on—especially the challenge of finding the real thing, instead of buying an adulterated fake olive oil from your corner grocery store—but the health benefits of consuming extra virgin olive oil are truly astounding. There are literally hundreds of high-quality scientific studies showing that this particular type of olive oil can suppress inflammation, help your heart, and even help control your weight. And the really good news? Authentic extra virgin olive oil is absolutely delicious.

Protein. The final macronutrient, protein, had enjoyed a run of great press for the last decade or so. Everyone from weight loss gurus to athletes have recommended dramatically increasing protein intake as a way to supercharge your metabolism. Protein is the "building block" used to create muscles and amino acids. It can be found in a variety of foods, including red meat, poultry, fish and seafood, and beans.

Protein itself is indeed a necessary part of any healthy diet, and according to the USDA, protein should be between 10 percent and 35 percent of an adult's

SUGAR: AMERICA'S TOXIC HABIT

There are a lot of reasons for America's (and increasingly, the world's) obesity epidemic, but I think one factor deserves special recognition: the incredible increase in how much sugar we are eating.

According to the American Heart Association, the average American adult eats a whopping 20 teaspoons of sugar every single day. The primary source of these sugars is sugary beverages, including sweetened fruit juices, soda, and non-soda sweetened beverages like flavored iced tea. Sugar comes in various guises, including the "ose" ingredients like dextrose, fructose, and sucrose; high fructose corn syrup; juice concentrates; honey; sugar; molasses; and syrup.

This extra sugar amounts to 230 extra calories a day for the average woman and 335 calories a day for the average man.[1] If you multiply that

---

1. http://www.heart.org/HEARTORG/HealthyLiving/HealthyEating/HealthyDietGoals/Frequently-Asked-Questions-About-Sugar_UCM_306725_Article.jsp#.VtckB5MrKcY

---

daily calories. The problem arises in exactly how people are getting their protein. The American diet is heavily skewed toward consumption of red meat and dairy, perhaps best symbolized by that most American of foods: the cheeseburger. But dinner isn't the only time we're eating red meat. Sausages and bacon for breakfast. Lunch meats and cold cuts for lunch. And spaghetti sauce or chops for dinner. When you consider that a single 8 oz. serving of beef could have 50 grams of protein—or about as much protein as anyone needs in a single day—you can see

out across an average week, it means that the average American woman is getting an extra 1,610 calories a week from sugar and the average American man is getting 2,345 extra calories every week. In other words, the average adult is eating almost an *extra whole day* in empty sugar calories every week!

No wonder people are gaining weight—but that's not the only issue related to extra sugar. Here are just some of the additional issues associated with eating too much sugar:

- Inflammation
- Increased risk of diabetes
- A diet deficient in calcium, vitamin A, and zinc
- Reduced fiber intake

I'm not saying you should never enjoy added sugar. But keep it in moderation, and whenever possible, avoid sweetened beverages and processed foods that are high in sugar. You'll enjoy the occasional sweet treat more if you can eat it without an extra helping of guilt!

that we are gorging on protein. And unfortunately, most of these protein sources are also loaded with unhealthy fats, especially saturated fat, which is found in animal products.

The Mediterranean Diet also includes plenty of protein, but it comes from lean and clean sources, such as lean poultry and especially seafood. Fish, especially cold water fish like salmon, is a great source of protein and healthy fats, including the critical omega-3 fatty acids.

By now, you're hopefully already seeing the outlines of the Mediterranean Diet come into focus. It's heavy on whole fruits and healthy vegetables. It relies on healthy fats like extra virgin olive oil. And it focuses on lean and healthy proteins like poultry and seafood. If you're a cook, you can no doubt already see the delicious potential of eating like this! Trust me, when the people in the Mediterranean basin developed their cuisine centuries ago, they weren't thinking about heart disease or obesity. They were using fresh and local ingredients to create delicious foods—and that's exactly what the Mediterranean Diet is all about.

And if you're not a cook, no worries. That's what SimpleMD is all about: bringing the profound and proven benefits of the Mediterranean Diet to everyone, no matter how busy you are.

MICRONUTRIENTS

Aside from macronutrients, the other component of a healthy diet are the micronutrients. Put simply, these are the vitamins and minerals. They are called "micronutrients" only because your body needs much smaller amounts of them to thrive, in comparison to macronutrients.

Micronutrients are obtained through a healthy diet or, when necessary and recommended by your doctor, supplements. Some of the major micronutrients include:

- Iron
- Calcium
- Vitamins (A, the B vitamins, C, D, E, and K)
- Magnesium
- Iodine
- Zinc
- Folate

Deficiencies in any micronutrient can lead to adverse health consequences. For example, iron deficiency (anemia) is related to cognitive problems, while iodine deficiency can cause goiter. Fortunately, true micronutrient deficiency in America is rare—no matter what the vitamin and supplement companies would tell you. Government agencies have launched ambitious programs to fortify table salt with iodine and flour with iron; both have been highly successful in reducing deficiencies in these two micronutrients.

While there are areas of the world with widespread nutrient deficiencies, the issue in America is usually *too much* of a good thing, not too little. Too many calories. Too much sugar. Too much saturated fat. Too much salt.

So, if you want to take a multivitamin every day to ensure you're getting enough of the vitamins and minerals, talk to your doctor about it. Most doctors have no problem with daily multivitamins or supplementation with some of the other micronutrients and healthy fats (especially the omega-3 fatty acids). But really, the best way to ensure you're getting everything you need is by eating a varied and colorful diet of whole and wholesome foods—exactly the type of menu you'll find on the SimpleMD Mediterranean Diet.

In the next chapter, we'll dig deeper into what makes the Mediterranean Diet so effective and I'll give you secret to making it so simple and convenient that anyone can enjoy its tremendous health benefits.

Chapter 3
Step Two: Rebuilding
Your Food Pyramid

AS A CARDIOLOGIST who has spent his life helping people prevent and treat heart disease, the Mediterranean Diet has been on my radar screen for a long time—but when it came to sitting down to create SimpleMD, there really was one moment that pushed me over the edge.

It started in 2013, with the publication of the first results of a Spanish study known as the PREDIMED study, or Prevencion con Dieta Mediterranea study. This original study was published in the prestigious *New England Journal of Medicine*, and I want to share what really caught my attention.

Conducted by a researcher named Ramon Estruch and colleagues, the PREDIMED study looked at the dietary patterns of 7,447 people aged 55 to 80 years old. Almost 60 percent of them were women. The group was carefully selected for their lifestyle habits. Once in the study, they were divided into three study groups, given thorough health exams and histories, and then tracked for almost five years. Two of the three groups ate a recommended Mediterranean Diet that included either a lot of extra virgin olive oil or mixed nuts. The third group was a control group that continued with their normal eating habits. There was no calorie restriction in any diet group, and no requirement for additional exercise.

The initial results were striking. People in the study who ate extra nuts and extra virgin olive had a 30 percent reduction in the risk of a cardiovascular event (e.g., heart attack). Further, the extra virgin olive oil group experienced a significant reduction in the risk of stroke.[8]

Fast forward a few years, as researchers continued to dig into the PREDIMED data, to an eye-catching study that was published in late 2015 on the benefits of the Mediterranean Diet and breast cancer.

As PREDIMED itself had shown, the Mediterranean Diet could reduce the risk of heart disease and stroke. This wasn't too surprising; there was already plenty of data showing that the Mediterranean Diet was good for your heart and arteries. But now a study came along that represented a paradigm shift in the way we think about nutrition and breast cancer. This new study, published in the *Journal of the American Medical Association*, looked at the rate of invasive breast cancer among women enrolled in the original PREDIMED study. And guess what? The study authors, led by Dr. Estefania Toledo, found that *a diet high in extra virgin olive oil actually reduced the risk of breast cancer.*[9]

This was the first randomized trial of any type showing that a particular diet could reduce the risk of breast cancer—and it all came down to extra virgin olive oil for the "primary prevention of breast cancer."

8. Estruch R, Ros E, Salas-Salvadó J, Covas MI, Corella D, Arós F, Gómez-Gracia E, Ruiz-Gutiérrez V, Fiol M, Lapetra J, Lamuela-Raventos RM, Serra-Majem L, Pintó X, Basora J, Muñoz MA, Sorlí JV, Martínez JA, Martínez-González MA; PREDIMED Study Investigators. Primary prevention of cardiovascular disease with a Mediterranean diet. N Engl J Med. 2013 Apr 4;368(14):1279-90.

9. Toledo E, Salas-Salvadó J, Donat-Vargas C, Buil-Cosiales P, Estruch R, Ros E, Corella D, Fitó M, Hu FB, Arós F, Gómez-Gracia E, Romaguera D, Ortega-Calvo M, Serra-Majem L, Pintó X, Schröder H, Basora J, Sorlí JV, Bulló M, Serra-Mir M, Martínez-González MA. Mediterranean Diet and Invasive Breast Cancer Risk Among Women at High Cardiovascular Risk in the PREDIMED Trial: A Randomized Clinical Trial. JAMA Intern Med. 2015 Nov;175(11):1752-60.

This is deeply exciting because it shows that the Mediterranean Diet isn't a one-trick diet. It's not "only" good for heart disease. In fact, the Mediterranean Diet is about glowing good health in every area of life.

THE MEDITERRANEAN-STYLE FOOD PYRAMID

Most of us are familiar with the government food pyramid, with its comfortingly familiar stacks of suggested food groups. When it was first introduced, the bottom layer of the food pyramid was built solely on grains (carbs), with the next layer up comprising fruits and vegetables. After we learned more about the dangers of bingeing on carbs, it was revised in 2005 and re-introduced as MyPyramid. This version was much less intuitive and featured colored wedges running up the side of the pyramid. Each wedge represented a different food group, including grains, fruits and vegetables, oils, milk and dairy, and meat and beans.

This new version of the food pyramid ran into immediate controversy from many quarters, including nutritionists who worried that it had been influenced by the food lobby, especially the diary and meat industries.

In 2011, only six years after MyPyramid was introduced, the government rolled out MyPlate, this time showing a plate divided into quadrants based on recommended food servings, with a separate glass for the dairy group. In this version, fruits and vegetables make up fully half of the plate, with the rest divided between grains and protein (e.g., meat and beans). According to the government guidelines under MyPlate, a healthy diet would comprise:

- O Vegetables: 40 percent
- O Fruit: 10 percent
- O Grains: 30 percent
- O Protein: 20 percent
- O Dairy: Unspecified, but daily

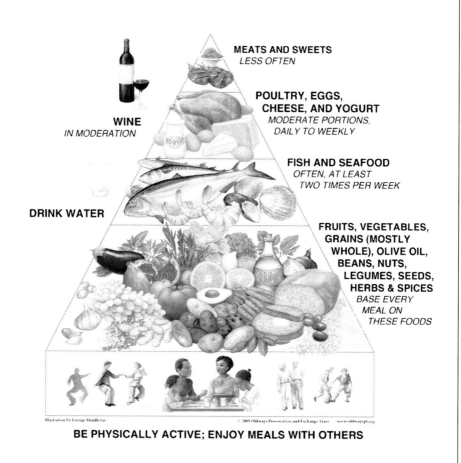

THE MEDITERRANEAN-STYLE FOOD PYRAMID
A Contemporary Approach to Delicious, Healthy Eating

MEATS AND SWEETS
LESS OFTEN

POULTRY, EGGS, CHEESE, AND YOGURT
MODERATE PORTIONS, DAILY TO WEEKLY

WINE
IN MODERATION

FISH AND SEAFOOD
OFTEN, AT LEAST TWO TIMES PER WEEK

DRINK WATER

FRUITS, VEGETABLES, GRAINS (MOSTLY WHOLE), OLIVE OIL, BEANS, NUTS, LEGUMES, SEEDS, HERBS & SPICES
BASE EVERY MEAL ON THESE FOODS

Illustration by George Middleton

© 2009 Oldways Preservation and Exchange Trust   www.oldwayspt.org

BE PHYSICALLY ACTIVE; ENJOY MEALS WITH OTHERS

This version was considered an improvement, but it still left a lot to be desired when it comes to following the scientifically validated principles of the Mediterranean Diet. For example, the government food plate makes no effort to distinguish between healthy fats and unhealthy fats. Likewise, there's little science backing up the idea that adults should be consuming any amount of dairy on a daily basis. Likewise, it only makes the most vague recommendations on the type of grains people should eat.

But I'm not here to critique the government's recommendations. Instead, I want to introduce you to a simple new food pyramid based on the Mediterranean Diet. This "new" food pyramid is actually more than a decade old, but it's still new to many people.

Let's take a look at some of the prominent features of this modified pyramid and how it fits into the Mediterranean lifestyle and the SimpleMD program.

Moderate Exercise is an everyday thing! But before you think, "Oh great, another doctor telling me I need to spend more time in the gym," think about the actual types of exercise that long-lived people in the Mediterranean basin get. They walk a lot. They play outdoor sports. They dance. All of this counts as healthy physical activity, and ideally, you should be getting 30 – 60 minutes every day of light to moderate physical activity.

Built on whole grains, vegetables, and fruits. The base of your diet is varied and healthy. It includes whole grains, beans, nuts, fruits and vegetables, herbs, and even spices. And don't forget the extra virgin olive oil, or EVOO! In the next section, I'll go into much greater depth about the incredible benefits of EVOO, but for now it's enough to know that this healthy and delicious oil should be a daily part of your diet.

Seafood is your friend. The American diet is heavy on poultry and red meat, including pork and beef. In contract, the Mediterranean Diet prefers protein from the sea. Why? For the simple fact that many types of seafood, especially cold-water fish, are loaded with healthy fats instead of the saturated fats found in red meat.

Poultry, cheese, eggs, and yogurt are preferred in limited quantities. Instead of breaking dairy out into its own group, the ideal Mediterranean Diet includes yogurt and dairy with poultry and eggs. If you have a real craving for dairy, I'd always recommend going with a low-fat or reduced-fat yogurt instead of cheese or whole-fat milk products. Yogurt is loaded with healthy bacteria that help keep your digestion moving and power your immune system. Eggs are also okay, especially as newer research is showing that the concern over cholesterol in eggs is overstated, but try to limit your consumption to 3 or 4 eggs a week.

GET A LOAD OF THESE NUTS

Any discussion of a heart-healthy diet wouldn't be complete without mentioning the powerful benefits of nuts. Packed with unsaturated fatty acids and antioxidants, nuts are frequently mentioned as a "superfood" in the same breath as kale, berries, and cold-water fish.

According to the Mayo Clinic, nuts are excellent for lowering "bad" LDL cholesterol, thanks to their high percentage of unsaturated fats, omega-3 fatty acids, fiber, vitamin E, amino acids, and plant sterols. In fact, up to 80 percent of a typical nut is healthy fat.

When it comes to what kind of nuts are best, most studies have focused on almonds and walnuts. However, it appears that any type of nut has health benefits. So feel free to enjoy roasted nuts as some of your daily dietary fat—and whenever possible, avoid salted, honey roasted, or chocolate-covered nuts.

Meat and sweets should be eaten sparingly. What does this mean? I'd suggest aiming to eat red meat once a week and switch out your dessert ice cream with fresh fruit.

Water and wine both make the list. Water is essential for life and good health, so you should be drinking plenty of water every day. There is a bit of controversy over just how much water people should be drinking. For years, the recommendation that people should drink eight 8-ounce glasses every day—known as the 8 x 8 rule—but newer research has called into question exactly how much water people should drink. Personally, I think the 8 x 8 rule is fine, if you remember to include ALL beverages in that rule. But if you only drink when you're thirsty, that's fine too, as long as you're drinking healthy beverages that aren't loaded with sugar and high-fat creamers.

As for wine, I'll discuss that in much greater detail in Chapter 5, but for now it's enough to say that wine, especially red wine, has very powerful health benefits that are unique.

Chapter 4
Step Three: The Absolute Importance of Extra Virgin Olive Oil

THERE'S A VERY GOOD REASON extra virgin olive oil (EVOO) is included in the very base of the Mediterranean Diet food pyramid. Put simply, it's an incredibly healthy fat that you should be consuming every day. EVOO is loaded with healthy monounsaturated fats and powerful antioxidants. In this chapter, we're going to take a look at what makes this oil so powerful—and the steps you need to take to ensure you're getting its full benefit.

HEALTH BENEFITS OF EVOO

EVOO is one of the purest and simplest cooking oils in existence. Without going into great detail, most of the vegetable oils in your local supermarket are highly processed and purified. They are built to last for a long time in your cupboard without oxidizing and without changing in their taste. To accomplish this, the oils are often extracted from their source (like soybeans or seeds) with solvents, then pasteurized at high temperatures, and treated with a procession of chemicals that might include phosphoric acid, sodium hydroxide, aldehydes, and others to achieve a bland, colorless, long-lasting product.

EVOO, on the other hand, is created from the first press of freshly harvested olives. Once the olives are pressed, the resulting juice is strained, bottled, and shipped, with all of its goodness intact. A good bottle of EVOO should actually taste like the olives it came from and it should be fresh. In many ways, this product is much closer to wine than to other cooking oils. Depending on where it's from and its quality, EVOO can be fruity, buttery and smooth, spicy, peppery, or just slightly bitter. In Italy, there's an entire profession devoted to tasting and rating EVOO for purity and flavor.

As you might imagine, this product is hard to produce—but the benefits are profound. In addition to the shocking study I cited earlier showing the EVOO can actually reduce the risk of invasive breast cancer, consider these findings:

- Extra virgin olive oil has been shown to protect the inner lining of coronary arteries and help lower blood pressure in women with high blood pressure.[10]
- A review of all the published benefits of EVOO found that it helped reduce inflammation in the coronary arteries, may help lower total cholesterol, reduced the formation of blood clots, and provided additional evidence that it supported healthy arteries.[11]
- EVOO has been shown to help prevent stroke in the eldery.[12]

---

10. Storniolo CE, Casillas R, Bulló M, Castañer O, Ros E, Sáez GT, Toledo E, Estruch R, Ruiz-Gutiérrez V, Fitó M, Martínez-González MA, Salas-Salvadó J, Mitjavila MT, Moreno JJ. A Mediterranean diet supplemented with extra virgin olive oil or nuts improves endothelial markers involved in blood pressure control in hypertensive women. Eur J Nutr. 2015 Oct 8.

11. Tovas MI. Olive oil and the cardiovascular system. Pharmacol Res. 2007 Mar;55(3):175-86. Epub 2007 Jan 30. Review.

12. C. Samieri, C. Féart, C. Proust-Lima, E. Peuchant, C. Tzourio, C. Stapf, C. Berr, and P. Barberger-Gateau. Neurology, Published online before print 15 June 2011

○ The Mediterranean Diet is the only diet scientifically proven to improve bone health and reduce the risk of hip fractures, according to the Journal of the American Medical Association in March 2016.

○ In lab studies, EVOO has been shown to slow tumor growth in colon cancer.[13]

○ Consumption of olive oil appears to support healthy brain function and might even protect against depression.[14]

EVOO has even been shown to benefit skin health. Leading dermatologists like Dr. Glynis Ablon, a professor at UCLA and a frequent expert on the TV show *The Doctors*, has long recommended the Mediterranean Diet for healthy skin, in part because of the EVOO.

Similarly, Dr. Leslie Baumann, New York Times best-selling author of *The Skin Type Solution*, writes that "your skin might just thank you" for consuming enough EVOO. She writes, "A report I authored in 2007 that was published in the *Journal of Pathology* discusses the role of antioxidants like vitamin E in contributing to radiant, younger-looking skin. The healthy amount of vitamin E found in olive oil has been shown to be successful in neutralizing free radicals and photoaging from UVA rays that damage skin cells, helping to maintain the appearance of youth.... In addition, olive oil contains linoleic acid, a component of skin that helps prevent water from evaporating (water is another substance

13. Terzuoli E, Giachetti A, Ziche M, Donnini S. Hydroxytyrosol, a product from olive oil, reduces colon cancer growth by enhancing epidermal growth factor receptor degradation. Mol Nutr Food Res. 2016 Mar;60(3):519-29.

14. Martínez-Lapiscina EH, Clavero P, Toledo E, Estruch R, Salas-Salvadó J, San Julián B, Sanchez-Tainta A, Ros E, Valls-Pedret C, Martinez-Gonzalez MÁ. Mediterranean diet improves cognition: the PREDIMED-NAVARRA randomised trial. J Neurol Neurosurg Psychiatry. 2013 Dec;84(12):1318-25.

EXTRA VIRGIN OLIVE OIL

5 Things You Need to Know

1. EVOO should be consumed every day as your primary daily fat.
2. The powerful benefits of EVOO are unique to authentic, first-pressed extra virgin olive oil.
3. Up to 80 percent of imported oil does not meet the legal definition of "extra virgin olive oil" and may not contain any olive oil at all.
4. Make sure you are buying the real thing, including the SimpleMD EVOO and products made with EVOO.
5. Aim to consume about 4 tablespoons a day, whether from SimpleMD bars, travel-sized packages, or a trusted supplier.

that promotes a youthful appearance). People who are deficient in linoleic acid can develop dry, flaky skin. Since linoleic acid is not produced naturally in the body, it needs to be supplemented in the diet or topically applied to the skin."

In fact, there is a convincing body of research showing that olive oil can be used as a lip moisturizer, after-sun treatment, deep hair conditioner, bath oil, and even may help prevent acne thanks to its high content of omega-3 fatty acids.

I could go on—there are almost 800 peer-reviewed studies on EVOO in the National Institutes of Health database—but you get the point. EVOO is unique among cooking oils for its ability to support a healthy heart, brain, vascular system, and newer research is even suggested reduce the risk of certain types of cancer.

So does that mean you should run out right now and buy the first bottle of EVOO you see on the supermarket shelves? Not exactly. Unfortunately, when it comes to EVOO, what you see isn't always what you get.

A NATIONAL EPIDEMIC OF FAKE EVOO

In early 2016, the respected news magazine *60 Minutes* ran a shocking story on Italian extra virgin olive oil. According to *60 Minutes*, the Italian olive oil industry has been thoroughly infiltrated by the Mafia. Yes, you read that right. Just like in the movie *The Godfather*, where the Corleone family was heavily involved in exporting olive oil, real-life Mafia figures have corrupted the Italian olive oil business.

How exactly? By selling fake product. According to *60 Minutes*, an astonishing 75 to 80 percent of Italian EVOO sold in the United States has been adulterated, diluted, or mislabeled, and does not meet the legal definition for EVOO. The most common form of fraud? Taking a standard oil, like sunflower oil, and adding chlorophyll and beta-carotene to make it look and smell somewhat like the real thing, *while in fact the bottle contains to no EVOO at all!*[15]

I was shocked when I saw this report. It's bad enough to defraud consumers by selling them a fake product, but when that product is also linked directly to better health, it takes on a new dimension.

So what can you do?

First, I would stress that there is a difference between other cooking oils, regular olive oil, and extra virgin olive oil. Only a true EVOO is loaded with the

---

15. *"Don't' Fall Victim to Olive Oil Fraud." 60 Minutes, http://www.cbsnews.com/news/60-minutes-overtime-how-to-buy-olive-oil/.*

ideal mix of antioxidants. Only a true EVOO provides the purest and best source of monounsaturated fatty acids. The fact is, there simply is no substitute for the real thing, both in terms of taste and health benefits.

At SimpleMD, we've been highly selective when it comes to our source of EVOO for our products. We can guarantee with 100 percent certainty that, when you buy a SimpleMD product that advertises "extra virgin olive oil," you are getting the full benefits of EVOO.

Second, when you buy EVOO, it's best to avoid the dozens of mass-produced Italian brands on the average supermarket shelf. If you insist on Italian, the best option is to buy directly from the producer and have it shipped to your home. However, this can be expensive—you might find yourself paying as much for EVOO as you would for a fine perfume or cologne!

A better option is to buy one of the up-and-coming California extra virgin olive oils, including the SimpleMD EVOO. Just like it did with wine decades ago, California is making a name for itself by producing authentic, high quality, and superior tasting EVOOs you can trust. These EVOOs have the benefit of being much fresher because they aren't stored and shipped overseas, so they are less likely to be rancid, oxidized, or fake.

HOW MUCH IS ENOUGH?

Once we agree that everyone should be consuming EVOO, the next question is: how much? A traditional Mediterranean-style diet calls for eating about eight to ten olives or ingesting three to four tablespoons of olive oil every day. The Food and Drug Administration recommends about two tablespoons daily. The PREDIMED study, the largest and most definitive scientific study on the benefits of olive oil, used four tablespoons a day as its benchmark. Because of the outstanding results in the PREDIMED study, I recommend four tablespoons every day.

Fortunately, extra virgin olive oil is so delicious that it's not hard to get those few tablespoons every day. You can use olive oil as a dipping sauce for fresh bread, in salad dressings, or in any of the recipes in the back of this book. We've also included EVOO in every SimpleMD product—five of our SimpleMD bars have about 1½–2 tablespoons. You can make up the difference either in salad dressings or as a dip for bread. We make it easy by offering travel-sized bottles of EVOO that easily slip into a purse or bag. Ingesting small amounts of EVOO throughout the day provides your digestive and circulatory systems with continuous protection against inflammation and oxidation.

When you're shopping for olive oil, you can always rely on our SimpleMD products to get the highest quality, authentic olive oil. If you're a grocery store, however, look for varieties that are cold pressed and organic, and specifically seek out those that are certified by the International Olive Oil Association or the California Olive Oil Council. High-quality extra virgin olive oil possesses a pleasant aroma, a deep green hue, and a delicious taste, often with a hint of peppery bitterness.

Chapter 5
Step Four: The Health Benefits of Red Wine

ONE OF THE EARLIEST CRITICISMS lobbed at the Mediterranean Diet was its inclusion of red wine on a daily basis. After being told for years that alcohol is empty calories, without any health benefits whatsoever, it was a shock to many people when the research started telling a different story. In this chapter, I want to take a look at the role that alcohol—red wine in particular—plays in the healthy Mediterranean lifestyle.

ALCOHOL: TONIC OR TOXIN?

The Mediterranean Basin, running from Spain all the way east to Italy and south to North Africa, has been a major wine-producing region for literally thousands of years. But it's only recently that scientists have begun to uncover exactly how the regular consumption of red wine has helped people in this area become among the longest living populations in the world.

I'll start with the alcohol itself.

Alcohol has been with us for thousands of years, and it has likely been controversial the whole time. Ethanol (alcohol) is a well-known toxin at higher concentrations. When you drink alcohol, it must be detoxified in the liver, which can take a serious toll over time. Excessive drinking is one of the leading causes of cirrhosis of the liver, an incurable, progressive, and frequently fatal liver disease. Excessive alcohol consumption is also known to impair judgment, reduce inhibitions, contribute to depression and other mood disorders, cause damage to unborn children, and is listed as a contributing factor in drunk driving accidents and domestic violence cases every day.

So there is no question that alcohol itself can be dangerous—but it's only more recently that researchers have begun to understand that, in moderation, alcohol has a number of health benefits. In general, "moderation" means 2 drinks per day for an adult male and 1 drink per day for an adult female. A drink is generally considered

SIMPLEMD'S SOURCE FOR THE BEST RED WINE

When we developed the SimpleMD line of Mediterranean bars, we knew we wanted to include red wine for its amazing health benefits, but we wanted to make sure we were sourcing our red wine from the best possible supplier.

Somewhat to our surprise, that led us to upstate New York.

According to research performed at Cornell University, red wines from New York State have the highest concentration of resveratrol in the world. Researchers announced this after comparing resveratrol content from more than 100 red wines from five states and overseas.

As a result, SimpleMD uses only New York State red wines in its product—so you can rest assured you're getting some of the best resveratrol possible.

12 ounces of beer, 5 ounces of wine, or a 1.5 ounces of a spirit. And in case you're wondering, you can't "save up" drinks over the course or a week. In other words, you can't skip drinking 6 days in a row and then binge with 10 drinks on a weekend night. Not only would that impair your judgment, it would result in a serious hangover and put a significant strain on your liver as it struggles to process all that alcohol.

In light of all these well-publicized negatives, what positives can there possibly be?

According to Harvard Medical School, alcohol in any form is known to help protect the heart, and moderate drinkers have lower rates of heart attack, strokes, blood clots, and overall death from heart disease. In fact, the overall risk reduction ranges between 25 and 40 percent.[16] That's a pretty significant benefit.

And just how does alcohol protect the heart? Moderate drinking has been shown to:

- Increase levels of "good" cholesterol (e.g., HDL cholesterol)
- Improve your body's sensitivity to the hormone insulin, which helps control blood sugar
- Reduce your blood's tendency to clot, which helps prevent the formation of clots that cause heart attack and stroke
- Reduce the risk of diabetes

When you put it all together, you come up with solid evidence that moderate and regular alcohol consumption is good for your heart, vascular system, metabolism and

16. "Alcohol: Balancing Risks and Benefits." Harvard T.H. Chan School of Public Health,

http://www.hsph.harvard.edu/nutritionsource/alcohol-full-story/.

others. This appears to be true no matter what type of alcohol is consumed—but that doesn't mean there isn't a superstar in the mix. Now let's take a look at red wine specifically and see why this particular beverage is linked to good health and long life.

RED WINE: POUR A GLASS OF HEALTH

Earlier, I talked about Blue Zones, or those areas where people seem to live the longest and have less disease. It's no coincidence that many of these are in the Mediterranean Basin, given that all the ingredients of a healthy, long life characterize this region. But now I want to turn to a different, and well documented, health phenomenon: the French paradox.

Researchers first noted this French paradox almost two centuries ago, when an Irish physician wrote that certain types of disease, including heart disease, are less common in parts of France (a region that shares many things in common with the Mediterranean Basin I've been writing about). Since then, numerous other researchers have confirmed that people who live in this part of France suffer from less heart disease and other types of disease. This is especially remarkable considering the typical diet in France: lots of butter and cream, with all of its saturated fats, and not especially heavy on seafood.

What was happening? How could this Western, industrialized country that thrived on a fat-laden diet have less obesity and heart disease than other countries with similar diets?

There appear to multiple factors, including the fact that people in this area tend to walk a lot—so they get plenty of exercise—but one thing stood out in particular: the French love for red wine.

If this is indeed true—if the French paradox is at least in part due to red wine consumption—what is it about this age-old beverage that gives it such special health-promoting qualities?

Perhaps not surprisingly, what makes red wine so powerful begins with the grapes. Wine grapes are full of powerful antioxidants called polyphenols. According to the *American Journal of Clinical Nutrition*, polyphenols are a particular type of antioxidant that is best known for preventing diseases like heart disease and cancer. They are commonly found in medicinal plants and are known to take an active role in enzyme activity and cell health.[17] It's also fair to say that research into polyphenols is still relatively new—this branch of science didn't really open up until the last 15 years or so, with an explosion of research into the varied benefits of polyphenols. Polyphenols can be found in green tea, coffee, herbs and spices, fruits, vegetables...and red grapes.

The chief polyphenol in red wine is called resveratrol. Resveratrol was discovered early in the 20TH century by a Japanese researcher, but it wasn't until a Harvard scientist published positive findings in the prestigious journal *Nature* in 2003 that global research on resveratrol really took off. Today, many of the major health benefits of red wine are credited directly to its high resveratrol concentration, and there are almost 8,000 studies on resveratrol alone in the National Institutes of Health database. Resveratrol has even attracted attention from life extension researchers, who believe that it may be able to extend cell life and someday be used to prolong human life.

While researchers are still digging to uncover exactly how resveratrol benefits human health, there is plenty we do know. Here is just a sampling of its proven benefits:

Heart disease. It helps protect the heart against ischemic heart disease. This is the most common type of heart disease and the cause of most heart attacks. There is some evidence that resveratrol might even be able to reverse existing heart

---

17. Manach C, Scalbert A, Morand C, Rémésy C, Jiménez L. Polyphenols: food sources and bioavailability. Am J Clin Nutr. 2004 May;79(5):727-47. Review.

disease. It does this by protecting the coronary arteries from damage caused by inflammation and oxidation.[18]

Cancer. Resveratrol, along with other plant chemicals, are known to target and disrupt the creation of cancer cells.[19]

Alzheimer's disease. Alzheimer's disease is one of the most pressing health issues facing our aging population. It is the primary cause of dementia and one of the leading causes of death in the United States. Exciting new research is showing that resveratrol can be an important part of a multi-faceted approach to treating and slowing the progression of Alzheimer's.[20]

Diabetes and metabolic syndrome. Resveratrol has been shown to modify certain brain chemicals that are closely linked to increased risk of obesity, diabetes, and metabolic syndrome, which are all closely related to increased risk of heart disease as well as a constellation of other health issues.[21]

Depression, autism, and bipolar disorder. Through its ability to support healthy brain function and regular neurochemicals, resveratrol can help prevent depression and bipolar disorder, and in some smaller studies, has been shown to reduce the risk of autism.[22]

18. Raj P, Zieroth S, Netticadan T. An overview of the efficacy of resveratrol in the management of ischemic heart disease. Ann N Y Acad Sci. 2015 Aug;1348(1):55-67.

19. Singh AK, Sharma N, Ghosh M, Park YH, Jeong DK. Emerging Importance of Dietary Phytochemicals in Fight against Cancer: Role in Targeting Cancer Stem Cells. Crit Rev Food Sci Nutr. 2016 Feb 6:0.

20. Singh AK, Sharma N, Ghosh M, Park YH, Jeong DK. Emerging Importance of Dietary Phytochemicals in Fight against Cancer: Role in Targeting Cancer Stem Cells. Crit Rev Food Sci Nutr. 2016 Feb 6:0.

21. Ibid.

22. Ibid.

MEDITERRANEAN DIET ALCOHOL RECOMMENDATIONS

- Adult Men: 1-2 glasses of red wine daily
- Adult Women: 1 glass of red wine daily

Note: You can get many of the same benefits from non-alcoholic red wine, although the alcoholic version is preferred.

This is just a fraction of the positive research on resveratrol, but it's enough to convince me that I can certainly enjoy my glass of red wine or two at night and feel good about it.

One last point I want to make about resveratrol and red wine: you can walk into virtually any health food store in the country and buy resveratrol supplements. Unfortunately, research suggests that resveratrol supplements are a less-than-ideal way to get its benefits. The problem is that resveratrol is very poorly absorbed into the bloodstream, so most of the resveratrol you would take in a pill form is washed out of your body without being absorbed. There are many scenarios where dietary supplements can provide support to your healthy lifestyle, but for now based on the totality of research we've reviewed, when it comes to resveratrol, it might be best to get it from red wine, which is a main reason why it is included in the SimpleMD methods and products.

DOES NON-ALCOHOLIC RED WINE STILL COUNT?

For people who don't drink alcohol, it can be frustrating to hear a doctor talk about the health benefits of red wine and wonder if they can achieve the same benefits. The good news is that non-alcoholic red wine contains many of the same antioxidants, including resveratrol, and might even have some benefits that the alcoholic version doesn't have.

First, resveratrol is derived from the skin of the grapes as they are crushed. In this sense, non-alcoholic red wine has the same exact health benefits of the alcoholic version.

Non-alcoholic red wine also typically has fewer calories. According to Ariel, a producer of non-alcoholic red wine, their non-alcoholic red wine has about one-third the calories of traditional alcoholic red wines, with only about 20 to 30 calories per serving versus 100. Non-alcoholic wines also have no risk of impairment and don't have the same dehydrating effect as regular wine.

Overall, I can confidently recommend non-alcoholic versions of red wine for their health benefits. Additionally, the amounts of alcohol content in our products is so low that we are not required to list it by the FDA.

Chapter 6
Step Five: The SimpleMD Rapid Weight Loss Program

I'M SURE SOME OF YOU skipped right ahead to this chapter to get to the good stuff! In previous chapters, I've worked to make the case that the Mediterranean Diet and lifestyle is one of the healthiest in the world. People who adopt this pattern of living and eating live longer, with less disease and greater health, than virtually any other populations on the globe.

Now, though, it's time to turn all this knowledge into practical, day-to-day action. I often tell people that, unless they are willing to move to southern Italy, they'll have to find a way to make the Mediterranean Diet work in their actual, hectic, American lives. And that's what this chapter is all about, so don't worry: I'm not going to advise that you cut back hours in the office, learn how to cook like an Italian grandmother, and source your fresh ingredients every morning from a village market. Instead, this is all about making the Mediterranean Diet work for you, in your current life. This is why we created SimpleMD, and I hope you'll see that it really can be simple.

DIETING VS. LIFESTYLE

Before I get started, I think it's important to touch a little bit on the difference between a diet and making a positive lifestyle change. Diets are something of a national obsession. Depending on which statistics you look at, as many as 1 in 5 Americans say they are on a diet on any given day, with most of them aiming to lose about twenty pounds.[23] This means every day, you can find tens of millions of Americans following whatever rules their weight-loss plan describes. They might be weighing foods, counting calories, figuring out food scores, cutting out whole food groups, or living on concoctions that came from our ever-more-popular juicers.

Unfortunately, research has also shown that the vast majority of these diets will fail. These numbers are even harder to pin down, but it's not uncommon to read that more than 90 percent of dieters will ultimately gain back any weight they lost.

So what's my point? Simple: *I am not advocating a "diet!"*

The SimpleMD philosophy rests on a few simple pillars:

1. You are not dieting. You are instead making a lifestyle change with long-term positive benefits.
2. You should enjoy — really enjoy — the food you eat!
3. Any changes you make should fit easily within your current lifestyle.

You'll soon see that everything I recommend falls in line with this philosophy. You don't need to count calories to be successful. If you like to cook, that's great—but if you don't, there's no reason to be stuck in the kitchen every day making every

---

23. *"Fewer people say they're on a diet." USA Today,*

   http://www.usatoday.com/story/news/nation/2013/01/07/decrease-dieting-weight/1814305/

meal from scratch and portioning it out in little plastic containers. And you should never go hungry, never feel like you're cheating yourself. In fact, you will probably feel better than ever before, while losing weight and making your doctor very happy during your annual check-ups!

CASE STUDY: SIMPLEMD BARS HELP MARNIE LOSE 21 POUNDS

Marnie came to me with significant concerns regarding her family's health. She was a 52-year-old divorced executive in a marketing firm who had a previous health scare with cervical cancer but was now in remission. Her HDL cholesterol was a few points below laboratory normal and her only son of 22 years was found to have an unfavorable cholesterol profile. She was considered pre-diabetic and was trying to lose 35 pounds to get to her ideal weight.

She was confused as to what diet to consider and concerned for her son's health as well. After hearing my perspective on the Mediterranean Diet and my passion for the SimpleMD products, she began adding the SimpleMD bars to her diet first as a complete meal replacement program. She quickly lost 21 pounds (60 days) and has maintained it every since. She soon recommended it for her son, a graduate student with questionable dietary habits.

Both mother and son lost weight and improved their cholesterol numbers. They both noticed improved energy levels and mood elevation. They now both carry SimpleMD bars with them so it's easy to make better choices during the day. They even carry a small amount of extra virgin olive oil so they can use it with either salads or with bread whenever they eat out!

GETTING STARTED WITH RAPID WEIGHT LOSS

The first step is always the hardest! If you've made it this far, then you see that eating a Mediterranean Diet will help you lose weight, feel better, reduce your risk of disease, and live longer. But remember: this isn't about starting a traditional diet. This is more about making changes in your lifestyle. So, if you know that one method works better for you than something else, feel free to adapt these principles to whatever works best for you. If you're the type of person who likes to make big changes all at once, go for it! Or if a more gradual approach works best, that's fine too. Take it one day at a time.

TO CLEAN OR NOT TO CLEAN?

Here's a simple piece of advice that many people find helpful when it comes to getting started with a new eating program: clean out your kitchen.

It can be wonderfully motivating to spend a morning or afternoon going through your kitchen and getting rid of all the bad-for-you foods that will try to derail your progress. Just get a large garbage bag and say goodbye to the cookies, chips, ice cream, old blocks of cheese, crackers, candy bars, frozen foods, and other assorted junk food that seems to accumulate in the kitchen.

If you find canned or boxed goods that don't fit your plan, you can donate these to a local charity or food bank.

For those of you with families, who might not be following your program, if you must keep some of these foods, it can help to isolate it in a single cupboard or crisper drawer in your fridge and declare this "off limits" for yourself.

Finally, remember that no failure is permanent. If you have a bad day and slip back to older eating patterns, don't dwell on it! Tomorrow is another day, so you can start again. Guilt and self-reproach are negative influences that will try to knock you off your new program.

NOW, LET'S GET INTO THE ESSENTIALS

Eat 4-5 Meals a Day. This is a critical change. Instead of eating two (or even one) big meal every day, aim for 4 or 5 meals every day. Typically this will include a breakfast, mid-morning snack, lunch, late-afternoon snack, and dinner. Ideally, your last meal should be eaten relatively early, by about 7 p.m., so your body has time to process and digest everything you've eaten that day.

This isn't about counting calories, but you should be generally aware of how many you're eating. In the first few weeks, I recommend that women aim for between 1,000 and 1,200 calories a day. For men, it's about 1,200 to 1,400. Again, spread these calories out throughout the day. This is important because it helps ensure that your blood glucose and insulin levels remain relatively stable, which prevents the familiar crash after eating a large meal. It also helps to blunt feelings of hunger and keeps your body supplied with a steady supply of nutrients.

Don't worry if this sounds like a lot of food preparation. It's perfectly fine to eat a SimpleMD protein bar for one or two (or even more) of these meals. Our SimpleMD protein bars are made with real EVOO and red wine and have less than 150 calories. And they're delicious! You can easily incorporate these into your program so you never have to worry about missing a meal.

In fact, in our practice, we often recommend that patients who need to lose a substantial amount of weight start with a month-long diet "bootcamp" of eating 4 – 5 bars a day, plus one meal consisting of a leafy green salad with EVOO and a lean protein. We've found it's relatively easy for people to follow, and it results in a period of faster weight loss while their metabolism resets.

Please note: this is not a long-term solution. I would recommend only following this type of eating plan for 30 days or less, and then making the transition into a more sustainable, long-term diet with three meals and two smaller snacks. The idea behind the 30 days is to kick start your weight loss and give you tangible progress toward your goal. In my experience, people are much more likely to be successful if they see results early on. It creates pride and a positive feeling, which is a much healthier mental space than self-doubt and recrimination.

Make Your Meals Mediterranean. This is the fun part! Once you're done with the 30-day induction period, you can switch to a diet of wholesome, fresh, and delicious foods at every meal. To make it easy, I've put together a list of 10 commandments to help you on your way:

1. Eat fresh fruit or vegetables at every meal, including breakfast.
2. Enjoy unlimited quantities of green, leafy vegetables.
3. Aim to eat a wide variety of colorful vegetables and fruits.
4. Consume EVOO with at least one meal every day, but two or more is better.
5. All grains should be whole grains.
6. Seafood should be your main source of protein.
7. Eat red meat no more than twice a month.
8. Dairy, especially cheese, should be eaten in limited quantities and not daily. Greek yogurt is the preferred form of dairy, as it contains lots of beneficial bacteria that help digestion.
9. Limit sweets and desserts

10. If you drink alcohol, enjoy 1 glass a day of red wine for women and 1-2 for men.

Hopefully you can see how much variety is possible when you eat like this. You have permission to eat unlimited and healthy vegetables and fruits, plus a whole world of whole grains and seafood. Eating should be a pleasure. People in the Mediterranean Basin aren't planning their meals by a chart, so I don't think you have to either.

I do recommend, however, eating at least one leafy green salad every day, ideally with a nice vinaigrette made from—you guessed it—extra virgin olive oil!

Drink Plenty of Water. I talked about the importance of drinking water earlier, but it's really important. If you want to follow the 8 x 8 rule of drinking eight 8-ounce glasses of water every day, that's fine. If you'd prefer to be more relaxed, that's fine too. Just make sure you're drinking lots of water. From a purely scientific point of view, your body is basically one large, never-ending series of chemical reactions, and all of those reactions take place in a solution of water. Water is essential for proper cell function and detoxification.

Get Some Exercise Every Day. Ideally, you should be getting around 30 minutes of light to moderate exercise every day. It's even better if you can get 60 minutes of exercise every day. This includes walking, swimming, time in the gym, bike riding—whatever physical activity you will actually do and enjoy. If you're already a gym rat, that's great...you're one step ahead of the game. If you're new to exercise, try to make it fun and keep it varied.

Get Enough Sleep. The actual number of hours of sleep an adult needs varies, but if you're consistently getting less than 6 hours of sleep a night, that's not good. Most adults need between 6 and 8 hours of good sleep every night to allow their body to heal and rest from the day's activities. If you have trouble sleeping, pay attention to your sleep environment. Avoid alcohol or food before bed. If you have a TV in your bedroom, turn it off well before it's time to go to sleep. Don't exercise within an hour before bedtime. Try reading a book just before bed to calm down.

Reduce Stress Where Possible. The body of research on the harmful effects of stress is impressive and should serve as a warning for most adult Americans. We know that stress causes inflammation, that stress is closely linked to the risk of heart disease and other serious medical conditions, that people who are under stress are more likely to be obese, and that overall mortality is negatively affected by stress. Some experts believe that our national epidemic of stress is the most serious health issue affecting our country.

Unfortunately, finding a way to de-stress can be dauntingly difficult in today's complicated world of 24/7 work. Hopefully, some of the measures I suggested above will help, especially the exercise. You can also try meditation—there are plenty of wonderful books on how to get started meditating—and some low-impact forms of exercise like yoga. Even carving out a little time to take a walk or sit outside and enjoy the sunset (with your glass of red wine!) can help reduce your stress burden.

If, however, you find that you can't escape stress, you can consider talking to a professional, who might be able to suggest stress-reduction techniques that will work for you.

MEAL DELIVERY SERVICES: WORTH A TRY

You might not be surprised to find out that my original interest in the Mediterranean Diet is personal. Before I sat down to develop the SimpleMD products, I switched to the Mediterranean Diet myself, hoping to accomplish many of the same things my patients are hoping for: weight loss, lower disease risk, overall improved quality of life.

Like most of you, however, I'm also a busy guy. Besides launching SimpleMD I'm a cardiologist with a busy practice. I'm a parent who goes to his kid's baseball games. And I like to enjoy myself every so often. As you can imagine, I don't have lots of extra time to spend in the kitchen whipping up 4-5 fresh meals a day. This means I do rely on my own SimpleMD bars to make sure I'm always eating right—and I have a secret weapon: Fresh Diet meal delivery.

Headquartered in Miami, Fresh Diet runs the largest national fresh meal delivery service. The founder, Zalmi Duchman, was introduced to me just as Fresh Diet was expanding across the United States. I was instantly interested. Fresh Diet specializes in developing and delivering meals that follow the principles of the Mediterranean Diet. I was asked to consult with them to help achieve the goal of being able to deliver three meals per day with a snack and a dessert that all met with the Mediterranean Diet principles. In a relatively short period of time, Fresh Diet was able to successfully deliver Mediterranean-themed meals to more than 10,000 customers per day.

GIVE FRESH DIET A TRY!

I find Fresh Diet so convenient, delicious, and healthy that I often recommend it for my patients. Hoping to introduce it to more people, we've partnered with Fresh Diet to offer 10 percent off to our readers and patients. To claim this discount, visit the Fresh Diet website at *www.thefreshdiet.com* and use the code SOFFERNY16 when prompted.

Whenever I return from a vacation, lecture series, or any type of travel, I sign up to their program for a few weeks. It's great. I find that the weight I inevitably gained while traveling quickly falls off and my eating pattern goes back to my healthier normal. In fact, if I am away for more than just a few days, Fresh Diet can deliver meals to most of the cities I visit in my travels.

Combine this luxury with our SimpleMD bars and I am never to far from making a "smarter choice." This truly adds a dimension of "reality and mobility" to the Mediterranean Diet that the world has never seen before.

Although there are other fresh delivery companies in the market, Fresh Diet has been very proactive in following the Mediterranean Diet on their menus and keeping their quality up. In fact, we were so impressed with Fresh Diet that I now recommend it to interested patients.

THE LAST WORD: IT'S WORTH IT!

In the preceding pages, I've tried to build a case for why the Mediterranean Diet and lifestyle is superior for your mental, physical, and emotional health. I've also tried to demonstrate how it can fit into your daily life...in other words, how it can be simple!

I hope it's clear by now that I don't believe in making dramatic life changes that are impossible to maintain over the long term and perhaps not even healthy. I believe the Mediterranean-focused lifestyle I've laid out in these pages is the path to a healthy balance, one that combines excellent and healthy food with good nutrition, adequate exercise and sleep, and relaxation. The SimpleMD program is all about living well and living long while following the scientifically validated principles of the Mediterranean Diet.

So, whenever you're ready, raise a glass of red wine in a toast to health and happiness!

THE SIMPLEMD JUMP START WEIGHT LOSS PLAN

Lose up to 15 pounds in just 4 weeks*

Are you ready to get started? Simply follow the instructions below and join the thousands of people who have gotten healthy the SimpleMD™ way! Remember, this is our "Jump Start" program and it is somewhat calorie restricted so it may be prudent to ask your physician prior to starting it. Also, we recommend using this program for up to 90 days and then periodically when needed to maintain your optimal weight. Once you have lost your desired amount of weight, begin to add back regular mediterranean diet meals and keep the SimpleMD bars available for when you need them.

We recommend that you consult your physician before starting this or any calorically restrictive program. This program is designed for a one month period; we suggest adding appropriate Mediterranean style meals once monthly goals have been achieved.

Note that this plan relies on eating five protein bar servings throughout the day. You can get these through our website, at www.simplemd.com. The introductory first-week box has 36 bars in a convenient package that can sit on your counter or travel with you. The box features three delicious flavors, a week's supply of EVOO, and all the happiness you need to lose weight, get healthier, and enjoy the journey!

*Individual results may vary.

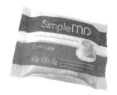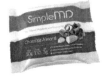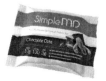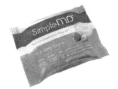

Dr. Soffer's Plan

Eat 1 bar at a time with water, preferably every 2–3 hours or when you feel hungry.

For breakfast

- Start with your first bar within an hour of waking up.
- Enjoy another bar between lunch and breakfast.

Throughout the day

- Drink at least 64 ounces of sugar-free, calorie-free liquids (i.e., eight 8-ounce servings) preferably water.
- Enjoy one bar for lunch and another for a mid-afternoon snack.
- No salads at lunch!
- See below, but you can split your dinner into two smaller meals if hunger is a problem.

For dinner

- 10-12 ounces of lean protein with non-starch vegetables, preferably 5 servings daily but a minimum of 3 servings.
- Choose from the lists below when picking your proteins

Acceptable proteins:

- Buffalo/Bison
- Chicken
- Turkey
- Fish
- Non-fat cheese
- Shellfish
- Egg whites/substitutes
- Tofu
- Ostrich
- Lean deli meat (turkey and chicken only)

Eat these proteins sparingly:

- Beef
- Pork
- Lamb
- Veal
- Salmon
- Egg Yolk
- Pompano
- Sea Bass
- Herring
- Mackerel

Eat as much of these as you want:

- Arugula
- Broccoli
- Cabbage
- Celery
- Green leafy vegetable

- Lettuce
- Mushrooms
- Spinach
- Zucchini

Limit or avoid these foods:

- Chickpeas
- Corn
- Kidney beans
- Legumes
- Peas

- Potatoes
- Pompano
- Sea Bass
- Herring
- Mackerel

Limit these to ½ cup:

- Asparagus
- Beets
- Brussel Sprouts
- Carrots
- Cauliflower
- Cucumber
- Edamame

- Tomatoes
- Eggplant
- Green Beans
- Onion
- Pea Pods (Snow and Sugar)
- Red & Yellow Peppers
- Squash

Foods may be baked, steamed, broiled, poached, grilled, and sautéed in limited amounts of extra virgin oil. No fats, no other oils, and no frying is permitted. Vegetables may be fresh, frozen or canned and eaten raw, steamed, roasted, grilled, sautéed with extra virgin oil, boiled or baked.

Salad dressings and other condiments used for your dinner meal should not contain more than 40 calories (i.e., 4 tablespoons of 10-calories-per-serving dressing). Use salt substitute when seasoning.

For dessert (pick one):

- One SimpleMD protein bar, heated for 10 seconds in a microwave
- Up to two individual servings of sugar-free Jell-O
- 1 sugar-free popsicle
- 1 dill pickle (if sweets aren't your preference)
- Celery

Ten Things to Avoid

1. Do not eat fruit or drink fruit juice (lemon and lime included). The natural sugar will cause hunger.
2. Do not eat bread, pasta, corn, rice or potatoes.
3. Use sugar substitutes only. No sugar or honey in any form.
4. Use breath strips and sprays only. Chewing gum and breath mints should not be used. They may trigger hunger.
5. For ultimate results, alcoholic beverages are not suggested except the minor amount already in the SimpleMD bars. Of course, when in the maintenance phase, we suggest 1-2 glasses of red wine per day. See our section on red wine.
6. Avoid personal trigger foods and shelf-stable foods (foods that are prepared with preservatives and do not require refrigeration).
7. Take one multivitamin a day.
8. If you are over 6'2", increase your bars cookies to 6 per day and if you are 6'4" in height increase your daily cookies to 7 per day.
9. Avoid fruit
10. Drink 8 glasses of water daily

See SimpleMD.com for more information!

Chapter 7
Recipes

YOU DON'T HAVE TO ENJOY COOKING to get the full benefit of the Mediterranean Diet—whether it's through our SimpleMD protein bars, a meal delivery service like Fresh Diet, or finding Mediterranean-friendly restaurants, there are plenty of convenience and easy ways to find great Mediterranean food. But if you do happen to enjoy cooking, you're in luck! The Mediterranean basin is home to some of the world's most celebrated and beloved cuisines, including Italian, Greek, southern French, Morrocan, and Spanish.

In the following pages, I've collected just a small sample of recipes from various sources that both satisfy the requirements of the Mediterranean Diet and are delicious as well. Once you get acquainted with these, feel free to experiment with these ingredients. There are also some excellent all-purpose cookbooks as near as your local bookstore that are loaded with more options.

And remember, try to incorporate authentic extra virgin olive oil into your meals wherever possible. The health benefits are profound and unique to extra virgin olive oil.

So, without further ado, here is a good place to start your journey into the healthy foods of the Mediterranean.

Breakfast

BREAKFAST COUSCOUS

Serves 8

INGREDIENTS

- 2 cups skim milk
- 2 tablespoons honey
- 3 teaspoons ground cinnamon
- 2 cups dry couscous

- ⅓ cup chopped dried apricots
- ⅓ cup raisins
- ½ cup slivered almonds

PREPARATION

1. In a saucepan over medium heat, combine the milk, honey and cinnamon.
2. As soon as it comes to a boil, stir in the couscous. Turn off the heat, cover and let stand for 5 minutes.
3. Stir in the apricots, raisins and almonds.

AVOCADO TOAST

Serves 4

INGREDIENTS

- 2 small firm ripe avocados, stone removed, peeled
- 80 grams soft feta, crumbled
- 2 tablespoons chopped fresh mint, plus extra to garnish
- squeeze of fresh lemon juice, to taste
- 4 large slices rye bread

PREPARATION

1. Place the avocado in a medium size bowl and mash roughly with a fork.
2. Add mint and a large squeeze of lemon juice, mash until just combined. Season to taste with sea salt and freshly ground black pepper.
3. Toast or grill rye bread until golden. To serve, spoon ¼ of the avocado mixture onto each slice of bread. Top with feta. Serve immediately garnished with extra mint.

PANCAKES

Serves 6

INGREDIENTS

- 1 cup old-fashioned oats
- ½ cup all purpose flour
- 2 tablespoons flax seeds
- 1 teaspoon baking soda
- ¼ teaspoon salt
- 2 cups Greek yogurt (plain or vanilla)
- 2 large eggs
- 2 tablespoons agave or honey
- 2 tablespoons canola oil
- Syrup, fresh fruit, or other toppings

PREPARATION

1. Combine first five ingredients in a blender and pulse process 30 seconds.
2. Add yogurt, eggs, oil, and agave and blend until smooth. Let batter stand to thicken, about 20 minutes.
3. Heat large non-stick skillet over medium heat. Brush skillet with oil. Working in batches, ladle batter by ¼ cupfuls into skillet. Cook pancakes until bottoms are golden brown and bubbles form on top, about 2 minutes. Turn pancakes over; cook until bottoms are golden brown, about 2 minutes.
4. Transfer to baking sheet. Keep warm in oven. Repeat with remaining batter, brushing skillet with more butter as necessary. Serve with desired toppings.

FRITTATA

Serves 6

INGREDIENTS

- 1 cup chopped onion
- 2 cloves garlic, minced
- 3 tablespoons extra virgin olive oil
- 8 eggs, beaten
- ¼ cup half-and-half, light cream or milk
- ½ cup crumbled feta cheese (2 ounces)
- ½ cup chopped bottled roasted red sweet peppers
- ½ cup sliced kalamata or pitted ripe olives, optional
- ¼ cup slivered fresh basil
- ⅛ teaspoon ground black pepper
- ½ cup onion-and-garlic croutons, coarsely crushed
- 2 tablespoons finely shredded Parmesan cheese
- Fresh basil leaves (optional)

PREPARATION

1. Preheat broiler. In a large broilerproof skillet cook onion and garlic in 2 tablespoons hot oil until onion is just tender.

2. Meanwhile, in a bowl, beat together eggs and half-and-half. Stir in feta cheese, roasted sweet pepper, olives (if desired), basil, and black pepper.

3. Pour egg mixture over onion mixture in skillet. Cook over medium heat. As mixture sets, run a spatula around the edge of the skillet, lifting egg mixture so uncooked portion flows underneath. Continue cooking and lifting edges until egg mixture is almost set (surface will be moist.) Reduce heat as necessary to prevent overcooking.

4. In a bowl combine crushed croutons, Parmesan cheese, and the remaining tablespoon of oil; sprinkle mixture over frittata. Broil 4 to 5 inches from heat for 1 to 2 minutes or until top is set and crumbs are golden. Cut frittata in wedges to serve. If desired, garnish with fresh basil leaves.

BANANA NUT OATMEAL

Serves 1

INGREDIENTS

- ¼ cup quick cooking oats
- ½ cup skim milk
- 1 teaspoon flax seeds
- 2 tablespoons chopped walnuts
- 3 tablespoons honey
- 1 banana, peeled

PREPARATION

1. Combine the oats, milk, flax seeds, walnuts, honey, and banana in a microwave-safe bowl. Cook in microwave on High for 2 minutes.
2. Mash the banana with a fork and stir into the mixture. Serve hot.

VEGGIE OMELET

Serves 4

INGREDIENTS

- 1 tablespoon extra virgin olive oil
- 2 cups thinly sliced fresh fennel bulb
- 1 Roma tomato, diced
- ¼ cup pitted green brine-cured olives, chopped
- ¼ cup artichoke hearts, marinated in water, rinsed, drained, and chopped
- 6 eggs
- ¼ teaspoon salt
- ½ teaspoon pepper
- ½ cup goat cheese, crumbled
- 2 tablespoons chopped fresh dill, basil, or parsley

PREPARATION

1. Preheat the oven to 325 degrees.
2. In a large ovenproof skillet, heat the extra virgin olive oil over medium-high heat. Add the fennel and sauté for 5 minutes, until soft.
3. Add in the tomato, olives, and artichoke hearts and sauté for 3 minutes, until softened.
4. Whisk the eggs in a large bowl and season with the salt and pepper. Pour the whisked eggs into the skillet over the vegetables and stir with a heat-proof spoon for 2 minutes.
5. Sprinkle the omelet with the cheese and bake for 5 minutes or until the eggs are cooked through and set. Top with the dill, basil, or parsley.
6. Remove the omelet from the skillet onto a cutting board. Carefully cut the omelet into four wedges, like a pizza, and serve.

LEMON SCONES

Serves 12

INGREDIENTS

- 2 cups plus ¼ cup flour
- 2 tablespoons sugar
- ½ teaspoon baking soda
- ½ teaspoon salt
- ¼ cup butter
- Zest of one lemon
- ¾ cup reduced fat buttermilk
- 1 cup powdered sugar
- 1 to 2 teaspoons lemon juice

PREPARATION

1. Heat the oven to 400 degrees.
2. In a medium bowl, combine 2 cups of the flour, the sugar, baking soda, and salt. Using a pastry blender or a food processor, cut in the butter until the mixture resembles fine crumbs. Add the lemon zest and buttermilk, stirring just until mixed.
3. Flour a surface with the remaining flour and turn out the dough; knead gently six times. Shape the dough into a ball and then flatten into a ½-inch-thick circle with a rolling pin.
4. Cut the circle into 4 wedges and then cut each wedge into 3 smaller wedges, yielding 12 scones.
5. Place the scones on baking sheet and cook for 12 to 15 minutes or until golden brown.
6. In a small bowl, mix the powder sugar and just enough lemon juice to make a thin frosting. Drizzle the frosting over the hot scones and serve.

Lunch and Dinner

GRILLED SALMON AND VEGETABLES

Serves 4

INGREDIENTS

- 4 tablespoons chopped fresh basil
- 1 tablespoon chopped fresh parsley
- 1 tablespoon minced garlic
- 2 tablespoons lemon juice
- 4 salmon fillets, each 5 ounces
- Cracked black pepper, to taste
- 4 green olives, chopped
- 4 thin slices lemon

PREPARATION

1. Prepare a hot fire in a charcoal grill or heat a gas grill or broiler. Away from the heat source, lightly coat the grill rack or broiler pan with extra virgin olive oil cooking spray. Position the cooking rack 4 to 6 inches from the heat source.

2. In a small bowl, combine the basil, parsley, minced garlic and lemon juice. Spray the fish with cooking spray. Sprinkle with black pepper. Top each fillet with equal amounts of the basil-garlic mixture.

3. Place the fish herb-side down on the grill. Grill over high heat. When the edges turn white, after about 3 to 4 minutes, turn the fish over and place on aluminum foil.

4. Move the fish to a cooler part of the grill or reduce the heat. Grill until the fish is opaque throughout when tested with the tip of a knife and an instant-read thermometer inserted into the thickest part of the fish reads 145 F (about 4 minutes longer).

5. Remove the salmon and place on warmed plates. Garnish with green olives and lemon slices.

TUSCAN WHITE BEAN STEW

Serves 6

INGREDIENTS

- 2 cups dried cannellini or other white beans, picked over and rinsed, soaked overnight, and drained
- 6 cups water
- 1 teaspoon salt
- 1 bay leaf
- 2 tablespoons extra virgin extra olive oil
- 1 yellow onion, coarsely chopped
- 3 carrots, peeled and coarsely chopped
- 6 cloves garlic, chopped
- ¼ teaspoon freshly ground black pepper
- 1 tablespoon chopped fresh rosemary, plus 6 sprigs
- 1 ½ cups vegetable stock or broth

PREPARATION

1. In a soup pot over high heat, combine the white beans, water, ½ teaspoon of the salt and the bay leaf. Bring to a boil over high heat. Reduce the heat to low, cover partially and simmer until the beans are tender, 60 to 75 minutes. Drain the beans, reserving ½ cup of the cooking liquid. Discard the bay leaf. Place the cooked beans into a large bowl and save the cooking pot for later use.

2. In a small bowl, combine the reserved cooking liquid and ½ cup of the cooked beans. Mash with a fork to form a paste. Stir the bean paste into the cooked beans. *(Continued on following page.)*

3. Return the cooking pot to the stove top and add the extra virgin olive oil. Heat over medium-high heat. Stir in the onion and carrots and saute until the carrots are tender-crisp, 6 to 7 minutes. Stir in the garlic and cook until softened, about 1 minute. Stir in the remaining ½ teaspoon salt, the pepper, chopped rosemary, bean mixture and stock. Bring to a boil, then reduce the heat to low and simmer until the stew is heated through, about 5 minutes.

4. Ladle the stew into warmed bowls and sprinkle with the croutons. Garnish each bowl with a rosemary sprig and serve immediately.

PASTA WITH SPINACH, GARBANZO BEANS, AND RAISINS

Serves 6

INGREDIENTS

- 8 ounces farfalle (bow tie) pasta
- 2 tablespoons extra virgin olive oil
- 4 garlic cloves, crushed
- ½ can (19 ounces) garbanzos, rinsed and drained
- ½ cup unsalted chicken broth
- ½ cup golden raisins
- 4 cups fresh spinach, chopped
- 2 tablespoons Parmesan cheese
- Cracked black peppercorns, to taste

PREPARATION

1. Fill a large pot ¾ full with water and bring to a boil. Add the pasta and cook until al dente (tender), 10 to 12 minutes, or according to the package PREPARATION. Drain the pasta thoroughly.

2. In a large skillet, heat the extra virgin olive oil and garlic over medium heat. Add the garbanzos and chicken broth. Stir until warmed through. Add the raisins and spinach. Heat just until spinach is wilted, about 3 minutes. Don't overcook.

3. Divide the pasta among the plates. Top each serving with 1/6 of the sauce, 1 teaspoon Parmesan cheese and peppercorns to taste. Serve immediately.

MEDITERRANEAN TUNA SALAD

Serves 3

INGREDIENTS

- 1 (12-ounce) can albacore tuna in water, drained and flaked into large chunks
- ½ cup thinly sliced red onion
- 2 celery stalks, thinly sliced
- 2 tablespoons coarsely chopped pitted kalamata olives
- 2 ½ tablespoons fresh lemon juice
- 1 tablespoon extra virgin olive oil
- ¼ teaspoon freshly ground black pepper
- ⅛ teaspoon kosher salt
- 2 large tomatoes, sliced

PREPARATION

1. Combine first 4 ingredients in a medium bowl. Add lemon juice and next 3 ingredients; toss gently to combine.
2. Serve salad over sliced tomatoes.

SHRIMP AND PASTA

Serves 4

INGREDIENTS

- 4 ounces whole-wheat bow tie or other pasta
- 2 teaspoons extra virgin olive oil
- 1 clove garlic, finely minced
- 8 ounces raw shrimp, peeled and deveined
- 1 cup frozen peas
- 8 ounces artichoke hearts, drained from can or thawed and cut into bite-sized pieces if frozen
- ½ cup thinly sliced green onions
- 3 tablespoons lemon juice
- ½ teaspoon ground black pepper

PREPARATION

1. Cook pasta according to package directions. When the pasta is done, scoop out 1 cup of the pasta water and reserve. Drain and rinse pasta.
2. Heat oil in a large skillet over medium-high heat. Add garlic and shrimp. Cook for 1 to 2 minutes, until shrimp turns pink.
3. Add peas, artichoke hearts and ⅓ cup of reserved pasta water. Lower heat to medium. Cover and cook for an additional minute.
4. Add cooked pasta, green onions, lemon juice and pepper. Toss to coat evenly.
5. Add more cooking water if the pasta is too dry. Serve

STUFFED PORTOBELLO MUSHROOMS

Serves 4

INGREDIENTS

- 4 (6-inch) portobello mushrooms, stems removed
- Cooking spray
- 1 cup chopped red tomato
- 1 cup chopped yellow tomato
- 1 cup panko (Japanese) breadcrumbs
- 1 cup (4 ounces) preshredded part-skim mozzarella cheese
- ¼ cup chopped fresh chives
- ¼ teaspoon salt
- ¼ teaspoon black pepper

PREPARATION

1. Preheat broiler.
2. Remove brown gills from the undersides of mushrooms using a spoon; discard gills. Place mushrooms, gill sides down, on a foil-lined baking sheet coated with cooking spray. Broil the mushrooms for 5 minutes.
3. While mushrooms broil, combine the tomatoes, panko breadcrumbs, cheese, and chives.
4. Turn mushrooms over, and sprinkle evenly with salt and pepper. Divide tomato mixture evenly among mushrooms. Broil 5 minutes or until cheese melts.

GREEK SALMON BURGERS

Serves 4

INGREDIENTS

- 1 pound skinless salmon fillets, cut into 2-inch pieces
- ½ cup panko
- 1 large egg white
- 1 pinch kosher salt
- ¼ teaspoon freshly ground black pepper
- ½ cup cucumber slices
- ¼ cup crumbled feta cheese
- 4 (2.5-oz) ciabatta rolls, toasted

PREPARATION

1. In the bowl of a food processor, pulse salmon, panko, and egg white until salmon is finely chopped.
2. Form salmon into 4 (4-inch) patties; season with salt and pepper.
3. Heat grill to medium-high; cook, turning once, until burgers are just cooked through (5-7 minutes per side). Serve with desired toppings and buns.

CHICKPEA AND POTATO HASH

Serves 4

INGREDIENTS

- 4 cups frozen shredded hash brown potatoes
- 2 cups finely chopped baby spinach
- ½ cup finely chopped onion
- 1 tablespoon minced fresh ginger
- 1 tablespoon curry powder
- ½ teaspoon salt
- ¼ cup extra virgin olive oil
- 1 (15-ounce) can chickpeas, rinsed
- 1 cup chopped zucchini
- 4 large eggs

PREPARATION

1. Combine potatoes, spinach, onion, ginger, curry powder, and salt in a large bowl.
2. Heat oil in a large nonstick skillet over medium-high heat. Add the potato mixture and press into a layer. Cook, without stirring, until crispy and golden brown on the bottom, 3 to 5 minutes.
3. Reduce heat to medium-low. Fold in chickpeas and zucchini, breaking up chunks of potato, until just combined. Press back into an even layer. Carve out 4 "wells" in the mixture.
4. Break eggs, one at a time, into a cup and slip one into each indentation. Cover and continue cooking until the eggs are set, 4 to 5 minutes for soft-set yolks.

FAVA BEANS AND PITA

Serves 4

INGREDIENTS

- 1-½ tablespoons extra virgin olive oil
- 1 large onion, chopped
- 1 large tomato, diced
- 1 clove garlic, crushed
- One 15-ounce can fava beans, undrained
- 1 teaspoon ground cumin
- ¼ cup chopped fresh parsley
- ¼ cup lemon juice
- Salt and pepper to taste
- Crushed red pepper flakes, to taste
- 4 whole-grain pita bread pockets

PREPARATION

1. In a large nonstick skillet, heat the extra virgin olive oil over medium-high heat for 30 seconds.
2. Add the onion, tomato, and garlic and sauté for 3 minutes, until soft. Add the fava beans and their liquid and bring to a boil.
3. Reduce the heat to medium and add the cumin, parsley, and lemon juice and season with the salt, pepper, and ground red pepper to taste.
4. Cook for 5 minutes on medium heat.
5. Meanwhile, heat the pita in a cast-iron skillet over medium-low heat until warm (1 to 2 minutes per side).
6. Serve the warm pita with the fava beans (either on the side or loaded up with the bean mixture).

LENTIL SALAD

Serves 6

INGREDIENTS

- 2 cups water
- ½ cup dry brown or red lentils
- One 14.5-ounce can chick-peas, drained and rinsed
- 3 Roma or plum tomatoes, chopped, or one 14.5-ounce can chopped tomatoes, drained
- ½ yellow bell pepper, chopped
- 1 red bell pepper, chopped
- 1 carrot, grated
- Juice of 1 lemon
- 2 tablespoons extra virgin olive oil
- ½ cup chopped fresh cilantro
- Salt to taste

PREPARATION

1. In a 2-quart stockpot, bring the water and lentils to a boil on high heat; reduce the heat to low and simmer for 30 minutes or until tender.
2. Drain any excess liquid.
3. In a serving bowl, mix the cooked lentils, chickpeas, tomatoes, bell peppers, and carrot.
4. Whisk together the lemon juice and extra virgin olive oil.
5. Stir the lemon vinaigrette into the salad, top with the cilantro, season with salt to taste, and serve.

MARGHERITA PIZZA

1 Pizza

INGREDIENTS - Pizza Dough

- One ¼-ounce package active dry yeast
- 2 teaspoons honey
- 1-¼ cups warm water (about 110 to 120 degrees)
- 2 tablespoons extra virgin olive oil
- 1 teaspoon sea salt
- 3 cups flour

PREPARATION - Pizza Dough

1. Combine the yeast, honey, and warm water in a large mixer or food processor with a dough attachment.
2. Let the mixture rest for 5 minutes to be sure that the yeast is alive (look for bubbles on the surface).
3. Add the extra virgin olive oil and salt and blend for 30 seconds.
4. Begin to slowly add 3 cups of the flour, about ½ cup at a time, mixing for 2 minutes between additions.
5. Allow the mixture to knead in the mixer for 10 minutes, sprinkling with flour if needed to keep the dough from sticking to the bowl, until elastic and smooth.
6. Remove the dough from the bowl and allow it to rest for 15 minutes under a warm, moist towel. Follow the pizza recipe for baking instructions. (*Continued on following page.*)

INGREDIENTS - Pizza

- 1 batch Pizza Dough
- ¼ cup flour as needed for rolling
- 2 tablespoons extra virgin olive oil
- ½ cup crushed canned tomatoes
- 3 Roma or plum tomatoes, sliced ¼-inch thick
- ½ teaspoon sea salt
- 6 ounces fresh or block mozzarella, cut into ¼-inch slices
- ½ cup fresh basil leaves, thinly sliced

PREPARATION - Pizza

1. Preheat the oven to 450 degrees.
2. Roll out the dough to ½-inch thick, dusting the pizza dough with flour as needed.
3. Poke holes in the pizza dough with a fork (to prevent crust bubbling) and bake it on a baking sheet or pizza stone for 5 minutes.
4. Remove the pan and drizzle the crust with the extra virgin olive oil and crushed tomatoes.
5. Top the pizza with the tomato slices and season with the salt.
6. Blot the mozzarella slices dry with a paper towel and lay them on top of the pizza in no exact pattern. Top the pizza with the basil.
7. Bake the pizza for 15 minutes or until the cheese is bubbling.
8. To brown the cheese, place the pizza under the broiler for 2 to 3 minutes if desired. Allow the pizza to cool for 5 minutes before slicing.

RICE PUDDING

Serves 6

INGREDIENTS

- ½ cup basmati rice
- 4 cups milk
- 3 tablespoons sugar
- ¼ cup raisins
- ½ teaspoon cardamom
- ¼ teaspoon cinnamon
- ½ teaspoon rose water (optional)
- ¼ almonds, chopped
- 1 tablespoon orange zest

PREPARATION

1. Soak the rice in water for 10 minutes and drain.
2. In a heavy saucepan, bring the milk and sugar to a low boil over medium-high heat.
3. Add the rice, raisins, cardamom, and cinnamon and simmer over low heat until thickened (about 45 minutes), stirring frequently.
4. Remove from the heat and add the rose water (if desired).
5. Combine the almonds and orange zest. Ladle the pudding into serving bowls and garnish with the almond mixture. Serve hot or cold.

GRILLED CHICKEN PANINI

Serves 4

INGREDIENTS

- 1 pound chicken breast
- ¼ cup balsamic vinegar
- ½ teaspoon rosemary, minced
- 1 clove plus 1 clove garlic, minced
- 1 teaspoon sugar
- ¼ teaspoon red pepper flakes
- 1 tablespoon extra virgin olive oil
- Eight ½-inch slices French or sourdough bread
- 2 tablespoons mayonnaise
- Eight ½-ounce slices fresh mozzarella or fontina cheese
- ½ cup roasted red bell peppers, jarred or fresh
- 8 leaves basil

PREPARATION

1. In a bowl, top the chicken with the balsamic vinegar, rosemary, half of the garlic, the sugar, red pepper flakes, and 1 tablespoon of the extra virgin olive oil.
2. Toss to coat. Marinate in the refrigerator for 30 minutes to 2 hours.
3. Preheat the oven to 350 degrees.
4. Bake the chicken for 20 minutes or until no longer pink on the inside.
5. Allow the chicken to rest for 5 minutes and then slice into ½-inch slices.
6. Combine the mayonnaise and remaining garlic in a bowl and spread ½ tablespoon of the mixture on the unoiled side of 4 slices of bread.
7. On top of the mayonnaise, layer 1 slice of the cheese, 2 tablespoons of the roasted peppers, 2 basil leaves, a quarter of the chicken breast slices, and another slice of cheese.
8. Top each sandwich with another piece of bread (oiled side showing).

   (Continued on following page.)

9. Heat a grill pan over medium-high heat.

10. Place one or two sandwiches in the pan and top with something heavy (such as a tea kettle filled with water) for 5 minutes on each side. Repeat with remaining sandwiches and serve.

CHICKEN SOUVLAKI

Serves 4

INGREDIENTS

- ½ cup (2 ounces) crumbled feta cheese
- ½ cup plain Greek-style yogurt
- 1 tablespoon chopped fresh dill
- 1 tablespoon extravirgin extra virgin olive oil, divided
- 1¼ teaspoons bottled minced garlic, divided
- ½ teaspoon dried oregano
- 2 cups sliced roasted skinless, boneless chicken breast
- 4 (6-inch) pitas, cut in half
- 1 cup shredded iceberg lettuce
- ½ cup chopped peeled cucumber
- ½ cup chopped plum tomato
- ¼ cup thinly sliced red onion

PREPARATION

1. Combine feta cheese, yogurt, dill, 1 teaspoon oil, and ¼ teaspoon garlic in a small bowl, stirring well.

2. Heat remaining 2 teaspoons extra virgin olive oil in a large skillet over medium-high heat. Add remaining 1 teaspoon garlic and oregano to pan, and sauté for 20 seconds. Add chicken, and cook for 2 minutes or until thoroughly heated.

3. Place ¼ cup chicken mixture in each pita half, and top with 2 tablespoons yogurt mixture, 2 tablespoons shredded lettuce, 1 tablespoon cucumber, and 1 tablespoon tomato. Divide onion evenly among pitas.

BABA GANOUSH

Serves 12

INGREDIENTS

- 3 (1-pound) eggplants
- ¼ cup fresh lemon juice
- 2 tablespoons extravirgin extra virgin olive oil
- 3 tablespoons tahini (sesame-seed paste)
- ¾ teaspoon salt
- ¼ teaspoon freshly ground black pepper
- 2 garlic cloves, peeled
- ¼ cup fat-free sour cream
- 1 (7-ounce) bottle roasted red bell peppers, drained
- 6 (6-inch) pitas, each cut into 6 wedges

PREPARATION

1. Preheat oven to 375°.
2. Pierce eggplants several times with a fork; place on a foil-lined baking sheet. Bake at 375° for 45 minutes or until tender. Cut eggplants in half; scoop out pulp. Drain eggplant pulp in a colander for 30 minutes. Place pulp in a food processor; pulse 5 times. Add juice and next 5 ingredients (through garlic), and process until almost smooth. Remove from processor.
3. Combine sour cream and bell peppers in food processor, and process until smooth. Swirl bell pepper mixture into eggplant mixture, if desired. Serve with pita wedges.

TABBOULEH

Serves 8

INGREDIENTS

- 1 ½ cups uncooked bulgur
- 1 ½ cups boiling water
- 1 ½ cups diced English cucumber
- 1 cup chopped fresh parsley
- 1 cup diced tomato
- ¼ cup chopped green onions
- ¼ cup fresh lemon juice
- 1 tablespoon extravirgin extra virgin olive oil
- ½ teaspoon salt
- ½ teaspoon black pepper
- 4 garlic cloves, minced

PREPARATION

1. Combine bulgur and boiling water in a large bowl. Cover and let stand 30 minutes. Drain; place bulgur in large bowl.
2. Add cucumber and remaining ingredients to bulgur; toss well. Cover and chill at least 1 hour.

HUMMUS

Serves: a lot

INGREDIENTS

- 2 (15.5-ounce) cans no-salt-added chickpeas (garbanzo beans), rinsed and drained
- 2 garlic cloves, crushed
- ½ cup water
- ¼ cup tahini (sesame seed paste)
- 3 tablespoons fresh lemon juice
- 2 tablespoons extra-virgin extra virgin olive oil
- ¾ teaspoon salt
- ¼ teaspoon black pepper

PREPARATION

1. Place beans and garlic in a food processor; pulse 5 times or until chopped. Add ½ cup water and remaining ingredients; pulse until smooth, scraping down sides as needed.
2. Chill overnight
3. Garnish with a lemon wedge and fresh parsley sprig.

KOFTE

Serves 4

INGREDIENTS

- ½ cup pre-chopped white onion
- ⅓ cup dry breadcrumbs
- ¼ cup chopped fresh mint
- 2 tablespoons tomato paste
- 1 teaspoon bottled minced garlic
- ½ teaspoon salt
- ½ teaspoon ground cumin
- ¼ teaspoon ground cinnamon
- ¼ teaspoon ground red pepper
- ⅛ teaspoon ground allspice
- 1 pound lean ground round
- 1 large egg white, lightly beaten
- Cooking spray
- 8 (¼-inch-thick) slices plum tomato (about 2 tomatoes)
- 4 (6-inch) pitas, split
- ¼ cup plain yogurt

PREPARATION

1. Preheat broiler.
2. Combine first 12 ingredients in a large bowl; stir until just combined. Divide mixture into 8 equal portions; shape each portion into a (2-inch) patty. Place patties on a jelly-roll pan coated with cooking spray. Broil 4 minutes on each side or until desired degree of doneness. Place 1 tomato slice and 1 patty in each pita half; top each half with 1 ½ teaspoons yogurt.

GREEK CHICKEN SALAD

Serves 4

INGREDIENTS

- 1 teaspoon dried oregano
- ½ teaspoon garlic powder
- ¾ teaspoon black pepper, divided
- ½ teaspoon salt, divided
- Cooking spray
- 1 pound skinless, boneless chicken breast, cut into 1-inch cubes
- 5 teaspoons fresh lemon juice, divided
- 1 cup plain fat-free yogurt
- 2 teaspoons tahini (sesame-seed paste)
- 1 teaspoon bottled minced garlic
- 8 cups chopped romaine lettuce
- 1 cup peeled chopped English cucumber
- 1 cup grape tomatoes, halved
- 6 pitted kalamata olives, halved
- ¼ cup (1 ounce) crumbled feta cheese

PREPARATION

1. Combine oregano, garlic powder, ½ teaspoon pepper, and ¼ teaspoon salt in a bowl.
2. Heat a nonstick skillet over medium-high heat. Coat pan with cooking spray. Add chicken and spice mixture; sauté until chicken is done. Drizzle with 1 tablespoon juice; stir. Remove from pan.
3. Combine remaining 2 teaspoons juice, remaining ¼ teaspoon salt, remaining ¼ teaspoon pepper, yogurt, tahini, and garlic in a small bowl; stir well.
4. Combine lettuce, cucumber, tomatoes, and olives. Place 2 ½ cups of lettuce mixture on each of 4 plates.
5. Top each serving with ½ cup chicken mixture and 1 tablespoon cheese. Drizzle each serving with 3 tablespoons yogurt mixture.

PITA WITH LAMB

Serves 4

INGREDIENTS

- 2 teaspoons extra virgin olive oil
- 1 tablespoon chopped fresh rosemary
- 1 teaspoon bottled minced garlic
- ½ teaspoon salt, divided
- ¼ teaspoon black pepper
- 1 pound boneless leg of lamb, cut into (¾-inch) cubes
- 1 ½ cups finely chopped seeded cucumber
- 1 tablespoon fresh lemon juice
- ⅛ teaspoon black pepper
- 1 (6-ounce) container plain low-fat yogurt
- 4 (6-inch) whole wheat pitas

PREPARATION

1. Heat oil in a large nonstick skillet over medium-high heat. Combine rosemary, garlic, ¼ teaspoon salt, ¼ teaspoon pepper, and lamb, tossing to coat. Add lamb mixture to pan; sauté 4 minutes or until done.

2. While lamb cooks, combine ¼ teaspoon salt, cucumber, lemon juice, ⅛ teaspoon pepper, and yogurt. Divide lamb mixture evenly among each of 4 pitas, and drizzle with sauce.

SCAMPI

Serves 4

INGREDIENTS

- 6 ounces uncooked angel hair pasta
- 1 teaspoon extra virgin olive oil
- ½ cup chopped green bell pepper
- 2 teaspoons bottled minced garlic
- 1 (14.5-ounce) can diced tomatoes with basil, garlic, and oregano, undrained
- ⅛ teaspoon black pepper
- 1 pound peeled and deveined medium shrimp
- ⅛ teaspoon ground red pepper
- 6 tablespoons (about 1 ½ ounces) crumbled feta cheese

PREPARATION

1. Cook pasta according to package PREPARATION, omitting salt and fat. Drain and keep warm.
2. Heat oil in a large nonstick skillet over medium-high heat. Add green bell pepper to pan; sauté 1 minute. Add garlic and tomatoes; cook 1 minute. Add black pepper and shrimp; cover and cook 3 minutes or until shrimp are done. Stir in red pepper; remove from heat.
3. Place 1 cup pasta on each of 4 plates. Top each serving with 1 cup shrimp mixture and 1 ½ tablespoons cheese.

ISRAELI COUSCOUS WITH CHICKEN

Serves 6

INGREDIENTS

- 2 ⅓ cups water, divided
- ½ cup sun-dried tomatoes
- 1 (14 ½-ounce) can vegetable broth
- 1 ¾ cups uncooked Israeli couscous
- 3 cups chopped cooked chicken breast
- ½ cup (2 ounces) crumbled feta cheese
- 1 cup chopped fresh flat-leaf parsley
- 2 (6-ounce) jars marinated artichoke hearts, undrained
- ¼ teaspoon freshly ground black pepper

PREPARATION

1. Combine 2 cups water and tomatoes in a microwave-safe bowl. Microwave at high 3 minutes or until water boils; cover and let stand 10 minutes or until soft. Drain and chop; set aside.
2. Place ⅓ cup water and vegetable broth in a large saucepan; bring to a boil. Stir in couscous. Cover, reduce heat, and simmer 8 minutes or until tender. Remove from heat; stir in tomatoes and remaining ingredients.

SCALLOPS AND ORZO

Serves 4

INGREDIENTS

- Cooking spray
- ½ cup pre-chopped onion
- 1 cup uncooked orzo (rice-shaped pasta)
- 1 cup fat-free, less-sodium chicken broth
- ½ cup dry white wine
- ¼ teaspoon dried thyme
- 2 tablespoons chopped fresh chives
- 2 tablespoons fresh lemon juice
- 2 teaspoons extra virgin olive oil
- 1 ½ pounds sea scallops
- ¼ teaspoon salt
- ¼ teaspoon black pepper

PREPARATION

1. Heat a medium saucepan over medium-high heat. Coat pan with cooking spray. Add onion to pan; sauté 3 minutes. Stir in pasta, broth, wine, and thyme; bring to a boil. Cover, reduce heat, and simmer 15 minutes or until liquid is absorbed and pasta is al dente. Stir in chopped chives and lemon juice. Keep warm.

2. Heat oil in a large cast-iron skillet over medium-high heat. Sprinkle scallops evenly with salt and pepper. Add scallops to pan; cook 3 minutes on each side or until desired degree of doneness. Serve with pasta mixture.

SPINACH, CHICKEN & FETA SALAD

Serves 4

INGREDIENTS

- ¼ cup fat-free, less-sodium chicken broth
- ½ teaspoon grated lemon rind
- 1 tablespoon fresh lemon juice
- 1 tablespoon balsamic vinegar
- 1 teaspoon sugar
- 1 teaspoon bottled minced garlic
- 1 teaspoon Dijon mustard
- 1 teaspoon extra virgin olive oil
- ½ teaspoon salt
- Cooking spray
- 1 pound skinless, boneless chicken breast
- ¼ teaspoon black pepper
- 1 ½ cups chopped red onion
- 1 ¼ cups (1-inch) pieces yellow bell pepper
- ½ cup (2 ounces) crumbled feta cheese
- 1 (15 ½-ounce) can chickpeas (garbanzo beans), drained
- 1 (7-ounce) package prewashed baby spinach

PREPARATION

1. Combine the first 9 ingredients, stirring with a whisk.
2. Heat a large nonstick skillet coated with cooking spray over medium-high heat. Sprinkle chicken with black pepper. Add chicken to pan; cook 4 minutes. Turn chicken. Add onion; cook 4 minutes or until chicken is done and onion is tender, stirring the onion frequently. Cut chicken into ½-inch-thick slices. Combine chicken, onion, bell pepper, cheese, chickpeas, and spinach in a large bowl. Drizzle vinaigrette over salad; toss gently to coat.

PASTA WITH SUN-DRIED TOMATO PESTO AND FETA

Serves 4

INGREDIENTS

- 1 (9-ounce) package refriger-ated fresh linguine
- ¾ cup oil-packed sun-dried tomato halves, drained
- ¼ cup loosely packed basil leaves
- 2 tablespoons slivered almonds
- 2 tablespoons preshredded fresh Parmesan cheese
- 1 tablespoon bottled minced garlic
- ½ teaspoon salt
- ¼ teaspoon black pepper
- ½ cup (2 ounces) crumbled feta cheese

PREPARATION

1. Cook pasta according to the package PREPARATION, omitting salt and fat. Drain through a sieve over a bowl, reserving 1 cup cooking liquid. Return pasta to pan.

2. While pasta cooks, place tomatoes and next 6 ingredients (through black pepper) in a food processor; process until finely chopped.

3. Combine tomato mixture and the reserved 1 cup cooking liquid, stirring with a whisk. Add to pasta; toss well to coat. Sprinkle with feta.

LINGUINE WITH PEAS AND CLAMS

Serves 4

INGREDIENTS

- 1 (9-ounce) package fresh linguine
- 2 tablespoons extra virgin olive oil
- 1 ½ teaspoons bottled minced garlic
- 3 (6 ½-ounce) cans chopped clams, undrained
- 1 cup organic vegetable broth (such as Swanson Certified Organic)
- ¼ cup dry white wine
- ¼ teaspoon crushed red pepper
- 1 cup frozen green peas
- ½ cup (2 ounces) preshredded Parmesan cheese
- 2 tablespoons chopped fresh basil

PREPARATION

1. Cook pasta according to package PREPARATION, omitting salt and fat. Drain; keep warm.
2. Heat oil in a large nonstick skillet over medium-high heat. Add garlic to pan; sauté 1 minute. Drain clams, reserving clams and ½ cup juice. Add reserved clam juice, broth, wine, and pepper to pan; bring to a boil. Reduce heat, and simmer 5 minutes, stirring occasionally. Add clams and peas to pan; cook 2 minutes or until thoroughly heated. Add pasta to pan; toss well. Sprinkle with cheese and basil.

CHICKEN SALAD PITA

Serves 6

INGREDIENTS

- 1 cup plain whole-milk Greek yogurt (such as Fage Total Classic)
- 2 tablespoons lemon juice
- ½ teaspoon ground cumin
- ¼ teaspoon crushed red pepper
- 3 cups chopped cooked chicken
- 1 cup chopped red bell pepper (about 1 large)
- ½ cup chopped pitted green olives (about 20 small)
- ½ cup diced red onion
- ¼ cup chopped fresh cilantro
- 1 (15-ounce) can no-salt-added chickpeas (garbanzo beans), rinsed and drained
- 6 (6-inch) whole wheat pitas, cut in half
- 12 Bibb lettuce leaves
- 6 (⅛-inch-thick) slices tomato, cut in half

PREPARATION

1. Combine first 4 ingredients in a small bowl; set aside. Combine chicken and next 5 ingredients (through chickpeas) in a large bowl. Add yogurt mixture to chicken mixture; toss gently to coat. Line each pita half with 1 lettuce leaf and 1 tomato piece; add ½ cup chicken mixture to each pita half.

SAFFRON FISH STEW

Serves 4

INGREDIENTS

- 1 tablespoon extra-virgin extra virgin olive oil
- 1 cup prechopped onion
- 1 teaspoon ground fennel
- ½ teaspoon ground coriander
- 2 garlic cloves, crushed
- 1 thyme sprig
- ½ teaspoon grated fresh orange rind
- ¼ teaspoon saffron threads, crushed
- 1 ½ cups water
- 1 ½ cups clam juice
- 1 (14.5-ounce) can diced tomatoes, undrained
- ⅛ teaspoon salt
- 1 pound flounder fillet, cut into (2-inch) pieces
- 1 (14-ounce) can great Northern beans, rinsed and drained
- Fresh thyme leaves

PREPARATION

1. Heat oil in a large Dutch oven over medium-high heat. Add onion, fennel, coriander, garlic, and thyme sprig; sauté 5 minutes. Stir in rind and saffron; add water, clam juice, and tomatoes. Bring to a boil; reduce heat, and simmer for 5 minutes. Stir in salt, fish, and beans; cook 5 minutes. Top with thyme leaves.

CHICKEN SHAWARMA

Serves 4

INGREDIENTS

- 2 tablespoons finely chopped fresh parsley
- ½ teaspoon salt
- ½ teaspoon crushed red pepper
- ¼ teaspoon ground ginger
- ¼ teaspoon ground cumin
- ⅛ teaspoon ground coriander
- 5 tablespoons plain low-fat Greek-style yogurt, divided
- 2 tablespoons fresh lemon juice, divided
- 3 garlic cloves, minced and divided
- 1 pound skinless, boneless chicken breast halves, thinly sliced
- 2 tablespoons extra-virgin extra virgin olive oil
- 1 tablespoon tahini
- 4 (6-inch) pitas, halved
- ½ cup chopped cucumber
- ½ cup chopped plum tomato
- ¼ cup chopped red onion

PREPARATION

1. Combine first 6 ingredients in a large bowl; stir in 1 tablespoon yogurt, 1 tablespoon juice, and 2 garlic cloves. Add chicken; toss to coat. Heat oil in a large nonstick skillet over medium-high heat. Add chicken mixture to pan; sauté 6 minutes or until browned and done, stirring frequently.

2. While chicken cooks, combine remaining ¼ cup yogurt, remaining 1 tablespoon lemon juice, remaining 1 garlic clove, and tahini, stirring well. Spread 1 ½ teaspoons tahini mixture inside each pita half; divide chicken evenly among pita halves. Fill each pita half with 1 tablespoon cucumber, 1 tablespoon tomato, and 1 ½ teaspoons onion.

Index

RECIPES

CPSIA information can be obtained at www.ICGtesting.com
Printed in the USA
BVOW01s0830160816

459125BV00005B/20/P